# INNER

# HUNGER

# INNER HUNGER

■

## A Young Woman's Struggle

### Through Anorexia

### and Bulimia

■

*Marianne Apostolides*

W. W. NORTON & COMPANY

NEW YORK · LONDON

#38043060

Copyright © 1998 by Marianne Apostolides

For information about permission to reproduce selections from this book,
write to Permissions, W. W. Norton & Company, Inc.,
500 Fifth Avenue, New York, NY 10110

The text of this book is composed in Electra
with the display set in Nicolas Cochin
Desktop composition by Gina Webster
Manufacturing by Quebecor Printing, Fairfield, Inc.
Book design by JAM Design

Library of Congress Cataloging-in-Publication Data

Apostolides, Marianne.
Inner hunger : a young woman's struggle through anorexia and bulimia / Marianne
Apostolides.
p.      cm.
ISBN 0-393-04590-0
1. Apostolides, Marianne—Health. 2. Anorexia nervosa—Patients—United States—
Biography. 3. Bulimia—Patients—United States—Biography. I. Title.
RC552.A5A66     1998
616.85'26'0092—dc21
[B]                                                                                         97–49805
                                                                                                  CIP

W. W. Norton & Company, Inc., 500 Fifth Avenue, New York, N.Y. 10110
http://www.wwnorton.com

W. W. Norton & Company Ltd., 10 Coptic Street, London WC1A 1PU

1 2 3 4 5 6 7 8 9 0

To those who have been through it,
and those who are still in it

# Acknowledgments

THANK you, Mom and Dad, for your caring and strength and love. Thanks also to my editor, Patricia Chui, to my agent, Flip Brophy, to therapists Preston Parsons and Amy Abern, and to my support system as I wrote this book—my friends Jenny, Anindita, Teddy, George, Sophia, John, Rick, Nicole, Mary, Rachel, Bonnie, Peter, Amber, Maureen, Jordan, Jerry, and especially Joel.

# Contents

# Introduction

I HAD binged the night before. When I woke up, a familiar pastiness glued the insides of my mouth. My eyes passed from one empty food wrapper to another—hollow packages of cookies, muffins, granola, bread—all lying in chaos on the floor. I was tired that morning. Tired of feeling disgust, anger, embarrassment; tired of lurching from starvation to binges to purges. I had felt that kind of exhaustion many times before.

I started dealing with the exhaustion in my usual manner: by focusing my mind, collecting my money, and buying food for another episode of bingeing. But as I stood in my dark apartment decorated with the remains of the binge, the tension I had held in my muscles released itself in tears. I dropped my money, took off my jacket, and turned on the computer. I didn't hesitate, I didn't look at the gray emptiness of the screen, I just wrote. All the emotions I had suppressed by means of diets and rules and binges and routines gathered in my body, moved through my fingers, and charged the computer with life.

The book I started that September morning in place of a binge took three years to complete. During those three years, I slowly let go of my eating disorder and filled my life and body with exploration, sadness, cycles, and desires—with the fullness of emotion and experience that comes with living. This is my story. While there are medical and clinical books on eating disorders, this is a personal book that takes you into the hate, fear, and confusion I felt during the ten years I was either anorexic or bulimic; and the ambiguity, energy, and expansion I felt as I released myself from those behaviors.

By sharing my story with you, I am trying to communicate directly with girls and women who have an eating disorder, and with their parents, mentors, partners, and friends.* To those readers with an eating disorder, I hope to connect with you on an emotional level. By connecting with you, I hope to offer some support as you establish new ways of dealing with yourself in your world. You are not alone in your behavior, and you are not forever locked into it. As you will see, a person with an eating disorder can find her voice, her balance, and her peace. To parents, mentors, partners, and friends, this book is a chance for you to understand, to feel the emotions your daughter or friend may not be comfortable voicing, to discover your role in helping someone you love deal with her emotional and physical pain.

To help you understand my experience as well as your own, I have included four clinical chapters: Chapter 1, in which I discuss the causes of eating disorders, and Chapters 9–11, in which I discuss the prevention and treatment of eating disorders. These chapters integrate extensive research, the wisdom I

*I have written this book specifically for females with eating disorders because I don't think I can properly speak to the experiences of males with anorexia and bulimia; boys and men, who make up about 10 percent of the eating disorders population, need a book directly addressed to them.

have gained through my own life, and the insight of Oakland-based therapist Preston Parsons. I am also including several definitions in this introduction so we can proceed through the book with a basic foundation of knowledge.

An eating disorder is not a disease, it is a set of behaviors that has no known specific cause. In clinical-psychology-speak, that means it is a "syndrome" with no known "primary etiology." The American Psychiatric Association (APA) didn't classify anorexia and bulimia until 1980, although the behaviors have been around for centuries. According to the APA's *Diagnostic and Statistical Manual of Mental Disorders IV*, a person with anorexia must weigh less than 85 percent of her minimum normal body weight, fear gaining weight, have a distorted body image, and be amenorrheic (without her period) for at least three consecutive menstrual cycles. Some anorexics are the "restricting type," which means they severely curtail their caloric intake. Others are the "binge eating/purging type," which means they regularly binge and purge, although they maintain an abnormally low body weight, unlike bulimics. A person with bulimia must have recurrent episodes of binge eating; purge the food through vomiting, laxative use, or strict dieting and exercise; assign undue importance to body shape and weight as a measure of self-worth; and binge and purge an average of at least twice a week for three months. Despite these definitions, I want you to know that you don't need to weigh less than 85 percent of your normal body weight or binge twice a week in order to address your eating behavior and its underlying causes.

Before moving on, I would also like to define four philosophies and movements that have shaped this book and my own worldview: confluent education, resiliency, harm reduction, and holistic therapy. Confluent education, which has much in common with holistic education, the Montessori and Waldorf methods, and Native American teaching, focuses on the education of the whole person. Those who practice these forms of teaching and learning work to develop students' cognition (mind), affect (feelings), and behavior in a way that promotes the growth of each individual. Resiliency argues that all people, even those in the worst situations, have an innate ability to survive and thrive. In its application to education in the schools, the home, and the community, resiliency focuses on the power of the life force within all individuals. Harm reduction maintains that people in difficult situations are best able to help themselves if they receive compassion, recognition for their knowledge and wisdom, and help in their effort to find their own path to change. Holistic therapies address the importance of dealing with the whole person, not merely the symptom of the person's problem, so that her/his mind, body, and spirit can work together to find balance, health, and healing.

As you read the following chapters, I hope those of you with eating disorders will feel connected or understood or strengthened. I hope the people who love you will start to understand and learn how to help. But in whatever way you read this book—with compassion, anger, fear, numbness, sadness, openness, love, hatred, or any combination of emotions—I hope it speaks to you with power and helps you nourish your own inner hunger.

# PART ONE

■

# I'm Hungry

# O N E

■

# The Causes of

# Eating Disorders

THIS chapter, based on my experiences, my research, and my conversations with professionals who work with adolescent girls, is a distillation of what I feel are the most important factors contributing to the prevalence of eating disorders among girls and women. If you want a comprehensive clinical overview of the causes of eating disorders, you can find it in other books. If you want a personal account from a woman who has been through the experience and the research, then read on.

In sweeping terms, eating disorders are caused by a person's need to find a way to function in her world when she can't do so in a healthy way. Instead of changing the way she relates to herself and her environment—her family, peers, community, and culture—she turns to food. Food lets her forget, provides the illusion of control, protects her from vulnerability. She creates rules instead of listening to the signals of her body; she focuses on numbers and routines instead of trusting herself to do and feel and be what is right for her.

There is no eating disorders gene, and there is no single experience or cultural pressure that causes someone to latch on to anorexia or bulimia. But in a more general way, a person's biology, experience, and environment can combine to make food/body manipulation the most effective stabilizer. The specific contributing factors discussed below do not in and of themselves trigger an eating disorder; rather, the trigger lies in the individual—in the way she experiences those factors given her biology, her prior experience, her environment, and the guidance she receives from others.

### The biological component of eating disorders

Our biology includes our innate physical and chemical makeup. Just as each of us will grow to an approximate height determined by our biology, each of us will grow to an approximate weight determined by our biology. The body tries to remain at that weight, called the "set point," by adjusting the level at which it burns calories: when a person's food consumption increases, so does her body's metabolism; when it decreases, her metabolism decreases as well.

While our physical beings are in part predetermined, so are our psychological beings. Everyone is born with a tendency to gravitate toward certain feeling states—melancholy, depression, optimism, obsessiveness, shyness, curiosity, etc. Some of us accept and explore those feeling states; others learn to handle them in a healthy way; still others try to blot them out through a destructive coping mechanism.

### Experiences and environment during childhood: Laying the foundations of eating disorders

So much of the way a person relates to herself, to other people, and to the world around her is formed by observing and participating in her family members' patterns of relating to themselves, to one another, and to the world around them. Certain common unhealthy family dynamics can lead to eating disorders.

By discussing these dynamics, I am not blaming parents for all the problems of their children. Parents have their own fears, desires, expectations, and coping mechanisms. They can't be blamed for those human qualities, just as people with eating disorders can't be blamed for theirs. But without knowing it and without meaning to, parents can foster an environment that makes their daughter vulnerable to using food/body manipulation as a coping mechanism. That lack of awareness is in part responsible for the development and continuation of their daughter's eating disorder.

Many parents have problems with food—they often diet, comment on their weight, scrupulously follow Weight Watchers' instructions. Through this behavior, they send skewed messages to their child about ways of dealing with food, hunger, body, and weight.

Other kinds of messages are sent by a family's approach to dealing with emotions: a girl might see her parents suppress their feelings or process them by fighting, drinking, turning sullen, etc. If parents don't give their child a comfortable space to process her own experiences and emotions—to cry or talk or argue—she may learn to suppress her feelings just as they suppress theirs.

Some girls learn that they must sacrifice certain aspects of themselves—their appetites, needs, feelings, and goals—in order to gain support, acceptance, attention, and love. These girls are called "people pleasers": they try to be everything to everyone. In doing so, they lose who they are to themselves.

During childhood, many girls learn that their bodies are not their own because they are being physically or sexually abused. The abuser—usually a relative or family friend—steals the girl's body, creating an association of the body with pain and terror, and a dissociation of the body from the mind and spirit. Between one sixth and one third of people with serious bulimic behavior wouldn't have experienced bulimia if they hadn't been abused as children, according to a recent study reported in the *American Journal of Public Health*.

The experiences of children in their environment beyond the family also shape their personalities. In certain common subcultures for girls—ballet, gymnastics, modeling, acting, etc.—a thin body is the standard for success and approval. Girls become aware of this standard through the comments of coaches, the gravitation of coaches toward those who have "ideal" bodies, and the example set by older girls thriving in these activities. When puberty makes a girl's body more curved and less like the subculture's ideal, that body becomes an obstacle—one that some try to eliminate through dieting.

The broader American culture also sends girls the message that they are valued for and judged by their body. A developing girl is encouraged to compare herself with an airbrushed, computer-enhanced version of a woman who fits the stereotypical, virtually unreachable ideal of the feminine: a boy's body—slim hips, thin arms, flat stomach—with large breasts and long hair. Most girls absorb those cultural messages and begin to resent the natural form of their body—a resentment that becomes more focused during adolescence and adulthood.

*Experiences in adolescence: Why food is an effective coping mechanism in the teen years*

A child's biology, experience, and environment shape her perceptions of herself, herself in society, and herself with other people. They shape the way she relates to the core of who she is. If that relationship with herself is strong, it can sustain her through the difficulties of adolescence. If it is not, she may need to protect herself through the relative safety of an unhealthy coping mechanism.

The nature of a girl's experience changes as she matures physically, emotionally, intellectually, and socially. But her ability to process that experience—an ability developed during childhood—may need to develop further before she can deal with her new reality. If she is left to swallow new circumstances without the proper tools to digest them, she may develop a coping mechanism that is unhealthy but necessary for her.

During adolescence, young people start developing an awareness of the power of their body and their sexuality. That power can be exciting, and it can be frightening. As a girl's body grows in ways she can't control—as her chest develops, her hips widen, her face softens—she typically doesn't see the beauty of that natural change, she sees only fat. Along with a changing body comes menstruation, with its messiness, discomfort, and unpredictability. During menstruation, a girl often feels as if something is hijacking her body, making it bleed. If a girl has had unwanted sexual experience through abuse, a changing body can mean greater fear of and hate for the body. A womanly, sexually mature body is seen as a dirty, dangerous object that attracts evil. By turning her anger, hate, and guilt inward, she hurts the body that has been the vessel for so much pain.

As bodies change, desires change. Instead of talking openly about those changing desires, our moral leaders often talk only about abstinence, the media flash images of sex to sell merchandise and entertainment, and our schools teach the statistics and mechanics relating to intercourse. Very few people talk with adolescents honestly and nonjudgmentally regarding their feelings about sexuality: their fears, desires, pressures, and responsibilities.

Given these changes and the lack of discussion about them,

food/body manipulation is a common coping mechanism. Anorexia stops a teen's body from becoming a woman's body. Despite her age, she again becomes flat-chested, her menstrual cycle is disrupted, the curves of womanhood sink inward, sexual desires cease to swell. If she cannot maintain her anorexia, she might start bingeing and purging—a further indication of her lack of control over her body and herself.

The hormonal changes that lead to physical maturity also lead to emotional maturity. Adolescents feel their emotions more deeply than they did as children: happiness, sadness, awkwardness, jealousy, loss, gain—adolescents feel them throughout themselves, throughout their bodies. A girl who hasn't had help developing a solid knowledge of herself—a sense of who she is, what she values, what she needs, and what she needs to avoid—can feel as if she is drowning in the waves of adolescent emotions. Anorexia and bulimia can calm the waves. Instead of feeling intense emotions, a girl can think about the number of calories in the apple she ate for lunch, or can plan the intricacies involved in executing and concealing a binge and purge. She can occupy her mind and time with the certainty of food, temporarily crowding out the uncertainty of emotions that come with living.

As the range of adolescents' emotions is expanding, so is the range of their intellect. Not only do they start thinking more conceptually and abstractly, they also start forming broad understandings of how they as individuals relate to other people and their environment. Most schools don't help students develop the whole of their intellect. They focus on rote learning, high achievement, and competition—known as the "masculine" part of each person's intellect—and largely ignore questions of interrelatedness and self-knowledge—known as the "feminine" part of each person's intellect.

Since our schools and society don't value or promote the feminine part of the intellect, adolescents often overdevelop the masculine part. To deal with that imbalance, some teens turn to eating disorders. An eating disorder can bring a girl out of her mind and into her body—she may stop studying, memorizing, and analyzing as she focuses on herself and the shape of her body; she may temporarily release herself from the stress of overachieving—the stress of trying to be the best student in class, the best student the school has ever had.

As their intellect matures, adolescents develop an awareness of themselves in their social world. Now that they see themselves as social beings, they need standards by which to measure whether they fit into their social surroundings. Those standards are provided by a teen's friends and other peers; subcultures she may join, such as a rock band or the student council; and the world of music, movies, magazines, and other media that tell girls what to look like, what to wear, what to say, how to flirt, how to be smart but not too smart, and on and on and on.

Girls with a strong sense of self are influenced by the media, and those who are vulnerable become overwhelmed by it. The popular media and those who create it are in part responsible for eating disorders because they create an atmosphere that encourages dieting, obsession about looks, and hatred of natural female bodies and beauty. But even though media images greatly contribute to the need for some girls to embrace anorexia and bulimia, eating disorders aren't imposed on us from the outside. The idea that we are drawn into self-imposed emaciation by pictures of models ignores the intertwined personal conflicts that cause eating disorders.

### The teen years may be the start, but they are not the end

The onset of eating disorders comes in waves: the first wave occurs at age thirteen, the second at age eighteen—the year most girls start college or leave school. Living away from home creates new possibilities and freedoms, but it also creates a vacuum of structure and rules. Those who don't know how to nourish their physical and emotional selves are susceptible to developing an unhealthy coping mechanism once they are away from the established dynamics of their family.

Eating disorders and disordered eating are two of the most common coping mechanisms on college campuses. Pressures surrounding body image and food are intense at college: the social scene often centers on big parties or the Greek system, which overemphasizes looks; the environment is extremely health-conscious in the purely physical sense of promoting high doses of exercise, but not in the fuller sense of treating the body, mind, and spirit with respect; and students often have to eat, in public, food that they have had no control over preparing. Those pressures have led to the high rates of eating disorders on college campuses.

Although most eating disorders begin while a person is in school, they do not necessarily end when a person leaves school at age eighteen to twenty-two or older. Once a person finds her coping mechanism in food and weight, she may have difficulty letting go of that mechanism, given her established patterns, the new wave of work and financial pressures, and the biological perpetuation of the eating disorder—the way the biochemical changes caused by the eating behavior create a physical need to continue that behavior.

EXPLORING THE WORLD—in other words, fully experiencing a range of environments with a range of people—means opening yourself to new pleasures, feelings, relationships, and beauty, as well as to moments of rejection, failure, and hurt. Each of us has her/his own individual reasons for feeling more comfortable exploring the world of food rather than exploring the world. Different biologies, life experiences, family environments, and cultural influences have shaped us into who we are at this stage in our lives. Right now, you may need a release in food. But you are forever evolving, expanding your world, changing the way you relate to yourself and others, changing your need for an eating disorder.

# T W O

■

# Family Dynamics:
# The Need Develops

MY family environment—an environment that taught me how to deal with myself in my world—was a cause of my eating disorder. That's not a judgment or a criticism; it's a fact to be accepted and processed, and it's a fact that helped me understand the path I took.

When my father, James, was eight years old, the Nazis invaded his hometown of Salonika, Greece. His father, Agamemnon, a prominent veterinarian who cared for cows, horses, and other animals important as sources of food and means of transportation, disappeared two years later. At the end of World War II, my father's family learned that Agamemnon had been captured and executed. Soon thereafter, my father left his homeland and immigrated to America, to be joined a year later by his mother and sister. I didn't know any of this history when I was a child zipping from tennis lessons to Broadway shows to soccer games, but I felt that history's presence in our house.

From the time of my father's childhood until now, he has prevented himself from feeling, expressing, and sharing his emotions with the people who love him. He has emotions like love, desire, pain, and despair, but he won't let himself feel those emotions; he pushes them down and focuses on the business of the day, which is running his veterinary hospital in suburban New York. My father's suppression of his emotions protected him during the times in his life when feelings would have overwhelmed him: when he wondered whether his father was alive or dead, whether the Nazis would ration enough food for the family, whether the immigration officials would let him enter the United States or send him back across the ocean. But while the suppression of emotions kept him safe, it also kept him emotionally unhealthy. For fifty years, my father has had to work to prevent his emotions from coming to the surface. His compulsive cleaning, obsessive exercise, and controlled eating have helped him achieve that goal.

I remember a cold morning on a family vacation to Maine when I was nine years old. The hotel room was still dark when I woke up to strange noises. I looked hard, squinted, and saw a shadow moving in the dark room. Dad was jogging in place. I had almost fallen back to sleep when I heard little grunts as he started doing sit-ups. A few hours later, while we were sitting at the hotel restaurant, my father scanned the menu and said, "This food sounds so good! But I'm not eating anything after this. This is it, this is my meal of the day." "Okay, this can be our big meal of the day, Jim," replied my mother, Frances, who was intent, as always, on pleasing us all. At the beginning of each vacation day, we would decide when we wanted to have our "big meal." If we wanted to have it at dinner, my father wouldn't eat any lunch. If we wanted to have it at lunch, he wouldn't eat any dinner. If we wanted to have it at breakfast, he'd pick at food for the rest of the day.

When we weren't on vacation, my father would push his

chair away from the dinner table each night, hold his stomach as if in bloated pain, and comment that he had eaten too much. It's as if he needed to justify having eaten a meal, having allowed himself to eat a whole plate of food. I never consciously registered his behavior as important. But I unconsciously got the message: control your food and your exercise, not by heeding your body's hunger and your desire to exercise, but by calculating calories and fat, and by obeying self-imposed rules. Control it.

My mother didn't control food. In her mind, she didn't control much, including the direction of her life. She is the intelligent, striking daughter of two immigrants from Greece. Her immigrant parents raised her with love and care and rules. Rule #1: You must go to Greek school to learn the language. Rule #2: You must marry a Greek man. Rule #3: You cannot go away to college. And on and on. The rules weren't horrifying in and of themselves, but they were part of a family system—a system that didn't include asking the children about their desires, opinions, and needs—that inadvertently stole my mother's power and confidence as a young woman.

My mother was a young woman when she rejected the offers of the University of Wisconsin and the University of Michigan to join their Ph.D. programs. Instead she worked in advertising and teaching for a while, knowing that when she got married she would quit her job and raise children. At age twenty-eight, my mother moved from New York City to the suburbs, becoming a suburban housewife who wasn't around the kind of cultural, political, and social stimulation she desired. She focused her energy on becoming a good wife and mother, neglecting her well-being as an individual. She sacrificed her own needs in order to meet the needs of her family. She forsook her own individual accomplishment and self-created happiness to live off the accomplishments and happiness of her husband and children.

When my mother wasn't preparing dinner, driving me to gymnastics practice, helping me and my brother with our homework, etc., she was busy doing volunteer work: on the phone as president of the women's auxiliary of a local hospital, doing bookkeeping for my father, participating on the evaluation committee for the high school student-exchange program. On the nights when she wore glasses and shuffled papers, she assumed an aura that attracted me. She was mysterious as she graded the papers of student-exchange candidates, her eyes moving like a typewriter across the page, her hand making authoritative marks in red pencil. She was confident as she tackled the bookkeeping, clicking fast on the adding machine, a pen horizontal in her mouth in case she needed to make notes or corrections. But in her work, as in the other aspects of her life, my mother was a caretaker. She didn't realize that even in that role, she could have asked someone to care for her, she could have shared her feelings and needs.

My mother didn't let anyone care for her the night her father died. Her face was red and her eyes sunken as she told us what had happened. My mother cried a lot after that night, but we never cried together. We never discussed my grandfather's sickness and we never discussed his death. My brother George and I didn't go to the funeral because my parents said we were too young, at ages ten and eight, and because they didn't want us to get hurt by being exposed to death, just as they didn't want us to get hurt by being exposed to any difficult situation. They wanted to protect us. But in protecting us, they sheltered us from experiencing, dealing with, and living through the full range of life.

In this setting, I looked to my older brother, George, as my role model. For twenty years, I thought his experiences were *the* experiences. When we were in grammar school, George was an all-star soccer goalie, the winner of the school backgammon tournament, an officer of the student council, a member of a pack of tight friends, and part of the gifted and talented program at school. In my mind, that meant I too had to be an all-star soccer goalie, the winner of the school backgammon tournament, an officer of the student council, etc. Even in grammar school, I felt I had a lot of work to do to measure up to my older brother. I got my first stress-related migraine headache in fifth grade.

ALTHOUGH I COULDN'T understand the causes or the depth of my parents' feelings when I was young, I absorbed their patterns of thinking, feeling, and acting—their inability to face, feel, express, and share deep emotions; my father's use of control, perfectionism, and exercise to deal with his feelings; my mother's unfulfilled desire to create an independent life based on her talents. I observed and internalized the way my parents and brother handled emotions, dealt with one another, and associated with our community. Those patterns, combined with my own intensity, the values of our society, and the pressures of adolescence, led me to develop an eating disorder.

I was in junior high now; my body was changing, and each day I was losing my sense of who I was. When I turned thirteen, my reality—what I believed to be right and reliable and true— shifted. My relationships changed, my desires changed, my body changed, my school changed. With everything changing, some of the patterns I had developed in my family environment—an inability to discuss uncomfortable issues, a fear of holding and feeling emotions, an unhealthy attitude toward food and exercise, a need and desire to be the best and match my brother's success—started to overwhelm me.

"Marianne, your dad's a veterinarian, right?" Alex looked over at me from his desk in health class.

"Yup." I felt privileged that he was actually talking to me.

"So I guess he grooms your hair then, right?"

The class laughed in unison, even my friends. I never went to health class without bringing my books for the next period. That way I could spend several minutes in the bathroom crying.

I had practically every class with Alex, Kevin, and Rich because we were in an honors program together. They discovered in me an easy person to mock: I didn't fade into the background like some of the other girls; I was naïve and self-righteous about drinking and fooling around; I spoke up in class, raised my hand, got good grades. A geeky prude—perfect fodder for Alex and company, who probably needed to pick on someone else to hide their own insecurities.

And yet while Alex mocked me, I wanted him, I fantasized about him. In my fantasy, I would open my locker to get some books and a piece of paper would float to the floor. I pick it up, curious. "Meet me tonight in the field. Don't tell anyone, just meet me. Alex." Heat fills my body. I look around. Alex is casually leaning his strong shoulder against a nearby locker. His shirt stretches across his muscled chest, and his clear eyes look at me, vulnerable. I meet him in the dark. Without saying a word, we kiss. We kiss hard and long.

*STOP! Get a grip, Marianne.* That's how I dealt with my fantasies—I dismissed them, denied them. I would be so *angry* at myself for feeling those feelings. So *angry* for being ugly and socially incompetent. How could I even think that I could be attractive to Alex! How could I be attractive to anyone, let alone Alex, Mr. Superstud Football Star, jersey number 34! I must be perverse! Disgusting! *Marianne, you're ugly. You've got ugly skin and ugly braces and frizzy hair. And he spends his time making the class laugh at you. He never even says hello in the hall. And you think he'll want you? Come off it, Marianne. Get a fucking grip.* Despite this reality, I couldn't let go of my dream that someday I could be the way I was supposed to be—like the cheery, fresh, I'm-so-cool-I-can-be-sexy-and-innocent-at-the-same-time girls on the cover of *Seventeen.*

The worse I was doing socially and emotionally, the better

George was doing. By the time we were in junior high, he seemed destined to become the high school's homecoming king, valedictorian, and class president. And he succeeded. At all three. I began to defer satisfaction, exploration, and experience by anticipating some future—some future that George had already reached—to bring me happiness. At the time my peers were exploring boundaries and living in the moment, I was looking toward that future instead of this present. I was always looking ahead and never looking around.

I had just finished the last leg of the 4-by-100-meter relay during track practice. When I was "walking it off," catching my breath, I saw Avery walk up to George on the neighboring field. Avery was thin and cute with short blond hair, a little nose, and a fragile smile that lit up her perfect pale skin. She was wearing a button-down white shirt and a long flowing skirt, the kind that makes many people look dowdy but made Avery appear the embodiment of femininity. George was wearing a grass-stained royal blue soccer goalie's jersey, the kind with the built-in elbow pads so he could heroically dive to stop a ball from getting into the goal. From where I was standing, I imagined that his face was wet with sweat and darkened with dirt. I watched the two of them and I wanted to be them: I wanted to be some pretty girl who could walk into a thick of guys and start flirting, I wanted to be a person my peers wanted to spend time with, like Avery wanted to spend time with my brother.

As I maneuvered through the new social terrain, the academic terrain was changing, too. In the transition to junior high, with harder classes and higher standards, I continued to strive to be the best. I had been put in special honors classes in seventh grade, and I felt that everyone expected good things from me—my parents, my teachers, my principal, me. I shook my head violently whenever I thought about what my parents, teachers, or even my brother would think if I got a bad grade. I couldn't handle the thought of letting them down. I had to keep working, keep practicing, keep performing, keep succeeding, so I wouldn't let anyone down.

Throughout junior high, I needed a safe space where I could feel and express my emotions, become aware of myself, and discover new paths, since the path I was on cut my body and spirit at every step. But since my family, community, and friends didn't help me create that safe space, I hid my emotions in anger.

After channeling that anger toward myself all day, feeding myself self-criticism and feeling the frequent flashes of embarrassment, I wanted to push the anger and hate onto another person for a while. My father was off the hook since he was a distant figure who purposefully wore his uniform and went to work each day, and since he was a disciplining figure who wouldn't let me direct my nastiness at him. My brother was off the hook because I worshiped him. So my mother—a woman who didn't go to work, had a weak sense of self, and thought she had the responsibility of making me happy and solving all my problems—received the literal and figurative punches of my anger. I wanted to make her feel the embarrassment and inadequacy I made myself feel. I wanted to control her because I couldn't control my life; to manipulate her by pretending I didn't love her, by denying her the love and acceptance I denied myself. My words told her I devalued her, hated her for not understanding my sadness, resented her for not having a job or serving as an example of the working woman I wanted to become.

My mother didn't back away from me or set boundaries for my behavior when I disrespected her. Since she thought she would be a failure if her kids weren't perfectly healthy and happy, my loathing just made her hover over me more, in an attempt to protect me from the pains of adolescence. She would tell me I was so pretty, so smart. She would tell me not to worry about anything, that I would always come through, that it would always be fine. I knew I was having problems, feeling unhappy, being mocked by my peers. But there was my mother telling me everything was just peachy. I felt that she was invalidating my experience, dismissing the power of my feelings. That dynamic made me hate her even more. And so we yelled at each other every day, starting when I was thirteen.

FOR ALMOST TWO years—when I was in seventh and eighth grades—I kept telling myself what I *should* be instead of letting myself find out who I was. Because I held my emotions inside me, my mind was always churning, twisting, spinning scenarios about how I had failed. I was always acutely aware of myself— my skin, my clothes, my laugh; my insecurity, my embarrassment, my nervous sweat. For a while, I wanted to be aware that I was in control of something.

"Not everyone can be beautiful, Marianne," Meredith said with sympathy in her voice, looking at me with her unblemished skin furrowed in seeming concern.

My throat tightened and I nodded my head as if to say, "Yes of course, I understand, Meredith, that's perfectly true." *Don't cry, Marianne.* I had no right to cry, no right to feel sadness or anger. I mean, she was beautiful and I wasn't, right? I was ugly and I should get used to it. *Get used to it, Marianne.*

I met Meredith at coed summer camp when I was fourteen. Camp was supposed to be amazing: this was my time to let go, have a summer romance, reshape myself into a fun, confident, popular girl. Now was my chance. Once again, reality was different from expectation. Changing my scenery wouldn't change me, but it would allow me to discover that I could use food to suppress my emotions.

There was a horde of us, pushing, waving money at the guy behind the snack bar. "I'll have, um, just the Oreos." He took my money, gave me the little blue package, and turned to the next teenage customer. I spotted Meredith at the center of a group of people, laughing, flirting, capturing the attention of the guy I was after. I didn't join them because I knew that if I did I would just stare stupidly as the conversation bounced from Meredith to the boys who surrounded her. So I turned away from the group and toward the narrow path leading to our cabins.

I moved fast up the path. No tears, no crying. Just fast up the path toward the cabin. I was tearing, ripping, biting the blue plastic package; I was eating with urgency, eating with violence, each little black cookie filling my mouth. Barely chewing, barely tasting, only taking, swallowing, breathing quick and shallow, I moved fast up the path.

When I got to my cabin I climbed into the top bunk, exhausted. I lay there grinding my teeth and vowed that I would never eat cookies again until I had lost weight. I told myself that food was my problem, my weight was the issue. If I lost weight, I would be okay, I would be popular, I would be happy.

That day at camp was the first time I sought relief from my emotions in food. I didn't cry, I didn't talk with a friend, I swallowed my emotions and ate. The eating disorder that started at camp would last for over a decade.

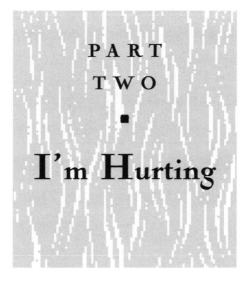

PART
TWO

I'm Hurting

# THREE

■

# Anorexic Adolescence

M Y anorexic headspace developed gradually in the months after my eating episode at camp. I started out like most dieters: by reading food labels, calculating the calories and fat in everything I ate, cutting out "nonbasic" foods—no snacks, no breads, no muffins, no sweets. After a couple of weeks, my clothes started to breathe a bit on my hips. I felt high, as if I were in an altered, excited state of mind. *I can do this!* I was taking control, making a change, getting sexy, becoming a woman.

"Here. Eat this." My mother slammed a huge plate of spaghetti onto the table. I stood in the doorway, my polyester volleyball uniform stuck to my sweaty body. I looked at the meat sauce sitting like vomit on the yellow pasta, and then at my mother, who was panting with anger, eyes big and mouth dry. While I was playing volleyball, my mother was planning how she would make me eat. She was trying to figure out how she could fix my problem of compulsive weight loss.

After five months of dieting, I weighed 109 pounds, even though my initial "goal weight" had been 118. I hadn't been happy when I was 118, so I had lowered the goal to 116, then 115, then 112. I had been exercising every day and progressively weaning myself off food: one day I'd use a teaspoon of salad dressing, the next week I'd sprinkle a couple of drops, the next month I'd decide I didn't need any at all—I'd decide plain lettuce tastes fantastic.

"Fine. Okay, Mom, I'll eat the spaghetti. Okay. . . . Just calm down." *Jeez, what is her problem? Fine. I'll just eat the food.* "Okay, Mom. I'm eating it. . . . Would you get off my case? . . . Just calm yourself." At that point in the anorexia, my fear of her panting and hysteria was sufficient to overcome my fear of the food.

My mother knew something was wrong with my mind-set, but she didn't know how to deal with it. She didn't know that "it" was emerging anorexia. Sticking a plate of food in front of my face was one technique for dealing with my anorexic behavior, but that technique wasn't very effective. It assumed that my problem was with food, not emotions; that my problem could be fixed by forcibly changing my eating patterns rather than helping me change my thought/feeling/behavior patterns.

One month after the volleyball game, I couldn't have eaten that plate of spaghetti. I would have screamed at my mother, scratched her arms, pounded up the stairs to my room. I would have done anything to avoid eating that food. By then I was fully immersed in my anorexic world with my anorexic thinking.

Anorexia infected every part of my life—my thoughts, emotions, dreams, desires, relationships, fears. I examined every potential activity in terms of the way it would affect my food intake. "Do you want to go to Karen's party tomorrow night?" *Will we have to eat dinner there?* "Do you want to go shopping?" *I can't go shopping yet. My gut is still too big.* "We're building the homecoming float on Saturday afternoon. Can you come and help?" *If I go, I can tell my mom I'm eating lunch there and I can tell the people there I'm eating lunch at home. So yeah, okay, I'll go.*

Everything related to food and exercise had to be the same from one day to the next. If I ate twenty flakes of cereal for breakfast one morning, I had to eat twenty the next day. If I walked up a flight of stairs five times on Monday, I became agitated if I walked up those stairs only four times on Tuesday. I told myself that any deviation from the routine would make me gain weight. I wasn't consciously aware of the real problem: that any deviation would take away all sense of control and order. So I walked up that flight of stairs a fifth time on Tuesday for no apparent reason.

The view of life through the prism of anorexia was distorting, but I needed that distorted world when the "real" world—the world of boys and dating and cliques and schoolwork—was more than my body and psyche could handle in a healthy way. When I got into the anorexic headspace, I was in a self-constructed, rational world where I didn't have to feel embarrassment, social failure, isolation, or self-hate. When I was thinking about weight control, I could wipe away emotion and go straight to cognition—to the hardness and reliability of calories, fat grams, numbers on a scale.

My dieting, along with my schoolwork, gave me a measure of comfort, an island of safety where I could rest when I was drowning in the social and emotional sea of ninth grade. On that island, my social and sexual development regressed. In more and more situations, I couldn't relate to my peers in their world because they were learning what it felt like to explore adolescence, while I was learning what it felt like to explore anorexia.

After a few months of lying to my friends when they called to ask me to join them at a party, the phone stopped ringing for me. I never faded from the group of friends I had established, in part out of inertia, in part because I always made myself available to listen to their problems. I could handle the role of mature confidante and later designated driver, but I couldn't handle the role of fun-loving friend. So as the phone sat silent on Friday and Saturday nights, I felt safe. I was free from the threat of gatherings with food and drinks and all those seemingly confident, beautiful, popular people. I was free from the threat of having sex with a boy. I was protected from rejection — from standing around and holding a beer but never drinking it, searching for Tim (the guy I had a crush on), watching Tim ignore me, wondering what to say, imagining other people looking at me and laughing, "What is *she* doing here? I thought she'd be at home doing homework or something. . . ." Because of my anorexia, I was free of all those uncomfortable feelings.

Anorexia also saved me from acknowledging that I was depressed at those parties, that I didn't fit in with that social circle. Instead of accepting that I was making myself unhappy by trying to squeeze into a group of people that made me uncomfortable, I wrapped my whole body around the excuse that I couldn't socialize because I wasn't thin enough. Once I got thin enough, I would be a calm, sexy, popular girl. If I could *only* lose a little more weight, if I could *only* flatten my stomach, then I would be welcomed into that world. After all, I was losing weight — I was doing something that all the girls were trying to do. So of course I would be socially accepted and comfortable soon, very soon. Change my body and I'll change my life.

In June of ninth grade, when I had fallen several pounds below the magical 100-pound mark, I tested my theory: I asked Tim, the cute class clown of junior high, to go to the junior high school prom with me. That morning, I put on a tight denim skirt and a crisp white shirt, top three buttons undone. I primed my hair, put on makeup. I looked good despite my gut, I thought. He would say yes despite my gut, I thought.

"Uh. That's nice of you. Really . . . nice. But, I . . . am . . . actually going with a couple of friends. Some guys . . . you know. . . ."

"Oh, sure. Well, okay. Well, maybe we can, like, dance or something when we're there?"

"Sure."

Two days later, Tim asked Tracy to the dance. Tracy had a squeaky laugh, a smooshed-in face, and a small, forceful body. She defeated me in an election for vice president of the student council that year, because she was popular. The teacher who ran the student council made me a nonelected officer because I was one of the few people who regularly attended meetings— something Tracy never did. I didn't like Tracy.

When I found out about Tim and Tracy, I skipped lunch and went to the library to do some work, but my mind kept drifting. *Damnit, I bet Tim's mocking me with all his goddamn friends. I bet little Tracy's mocking me, the little . . . Marianne, what were you thinking? How could you even ask him? You've liked him all year, and he obviously thinks you're a fucking geek, so why did you ask? Oh, Marianne, you are so, so stupid. . . .*

I escaped the self-denigration by counting calories. *I have to lose weight before the prom. So, okay, so what did I eat today? Cereal, 300 calories; slice of orange, 50 calories; apple, 100. But, wait, that was a big apple. So, okay, so 200 calories. So that's 550. Plus a cracker. Okay, so 700 calories. Shit, okay, so . . . okay, so I'll have a small dinner. Fine. Okay, back to work.* Four minutes later, I would do the same thing, overestimating the number of calories to make sure I didn't mistakenly eat too much. The calorie counting became automatic, not only when I felt a self-hating monologue building, but when I moved through my day. Calorie calculation was the first thing I did when I woke up, when I saw a plate of food, when I got dressed; it was the last thing I did when I lay in bed at night. Count and calculate. Over and over and over.

After dinner that night, I weighed myself: 94 pounds. *Okay, 94 is okay. So I lost a little. Good. But the prom is coming up and I want Tim to be pissed that he went with Tracy instead of me. So I'll do some more sit-ups. Then I'll do homework. Good, okay, good.* . . . Despite the monologue in my mind, I couldn't totally avoid my feelings as I lay in bed. I got angry at myself for starting to cry. I wanted to stop all feeling—to stop the aloneness and awkwardness. I clenched my jaw hard, ran my hand over my ribs, and played with thoughts of calories and weight.

I was asleep before 10 P.M. that night. That was usual for me: I had no energy to stay awake because I didn't feed myself. As I slept, I dreamed about food—towering boxes of cereal and big, chewy loaves of bread. Even though I rejected food, my body needed food, my emotions centered on food, and my mind thought about food constantly. Food fascinated, repulsed, and attracted me. It was my obsession. When I finished an apple, I'd start thinking about the lettuce I'd have at lunch. When I finished the lettuce, I'd start thinking about the chicken I'd have at dinner. When I finished the chicken, I'd start thinking about the apple I'd have at breakfast. With food so present in my thoughts, it was often present in my dreams.

I also dreamed about getting sick. In one dream, I am in a hospital room lying in bed. The lights are diffuse but somehow bright. The room is filled with people crying and talking to me. *I miss you, Marianne.* . . . *I hope you get better soon, Marianne.* . . . *Can we do anything for you, Marianne?* . . . *We were all talking about you, it's so awful what happened, we hope you get better, Marianne.* . . . Sometimes I dreamed I was in the hospital after being hit by a car as I bravely pushed someone to safety. Sometimes I dreamed I was there after attempting to commit suicide. In those dreams, Alex and Tim were at my bedside. They were crying, telling me they were sorry for the way they had treated me, telling me they wanted me to get better. . . .

While I dreamed of being the victim, I was making myself a victim through my starvation. Since I didn't feel capable of asserting myself in a positive way, I subconsciously "asserted" myself by becoming an emaciated, unhealthy, fragile girl. I got sick as a means of making people recognize that I had value. That strategy worked in my dreams, when Alex and his friends visited me in the hospital, gave me attention and compassion, went out of their way to accept me and to make me feel comfortable. But it didn't work in real life. No matter how much weight I lost, I didn't feel accepted by my peers and I didn't feel valued as a person.

Dreams of food and sickness overtook dreams of sensuality and sexuality. Through my anorexia, I turned my body back into that of a child—no more breasts or hips, no more period or sexual desires, no more masturbation. I chose to cut off the sensual signals my body sent me—the desire to enjoy food and touch and the curves of my body. By doing so, I cut off the sensual signals my body sent other people: my words and laugh were halting, my hair fell flat around my hollow face, my chest sank in and my bones jutted out, my skin glowed pasty white.

Even though I stopped sensing the emerging desires and power of my body, I still wanted some guy to like me and ask me out. But that desire wasn't something I felt in my body, it was something I thought in my mind. It was a desire for social acceptance, not a desire for the sweet anticipation or fantastic otherness of sensuality. When I became anorexic, that sweetness was gone.

BEFORE I STARTED dieting, I was aware on some basic, unconscious level of the need to exercise and to balance my intake of proteins, carbohydrates, and fats. My body indicated when it wanted to eat and when it was satisfied; it indicated when it wanted to exercise and when it needed to rest. But now I was ignoring my body's signals of hunger and satiation; I was letting my mind tell me when to eat and when to exercise. My mind said I needed to achieve my goal weight, wear size 2 pants, eat 600 to 1,000 calories a day, exercise sixty minutes daily, consume zero grams of fat. I no longer *felt* my body—no longer listened to it, sensed an impulse, and acted on that impulse. Now I *thought* about my body—devised a routine, calculated, measured its worth in numbers. The overthinking created static that let me ignore my agitated emotions, tired legs, and hollow stomach.

In my anorexic world, my body wasn't something I owned or enjoyed. I wasn't able to feel strong when playing sports, feel pretty when dressing up, feel sexy when fantasizing. My body was for other people to judge and take. As such, I had to make it worthy of being judged and taken. In my mind, it rarely was. I stripped down each night, weighed myself, checked myself in the mirror. I was happy about how much weight I had lost, but I wasn't happy about how I looked. At those times when I was most agitated, I looked at the reflection of my emaciated body and saw a big belly instead of the ridges of my rib cage. *Look at that gut. Look! It sticks out. Like a blob! It hangs out of you like a huge blob! I need to get rid of it. Get rid of it!* No matter how much weight I lost, I still had a gut, I still had a part of my body that wasn't flat and hard, I still had to diet.

But at those times when I was most calm, I realized I was too thin. I didn't realize that I was sick-looking or emaciated, with my skin clinging to my bones. But I knew I was too thin. "Hey, Susan, do I look too thin to you?" Susan was my gymnastics coach. She had long, thin legs—the kind of legs where the thighs are no thicker than the calves.

"No. I think you're fine." Great. I was fine. No need to worry.

Later that afternoon, Susan was spotting me as I practiced my vault. I ran hard, aced the springboard, held my body tight, and landed on the mat with a couple of hops. *Come on, Marianne! Stick the landing!* I was annoyed with myself.

"Marianne, maybe you *should* put on a little weight." It was Susan. She didn't comment on my vault. "Oh . . . you think so? Maybe, like, one or two pounds?" "Well, yeah. . . . Maybe four or five." *Okay. Four or five pounds. Well, maybe I'll just gain one or two, that'll be enough.* I was a little worried about having to gain weight, but I trusted Susan. She was my gymnastics coach, and she was thin herself. Since *she* was telling me I could gain a couple of pounds and still look okay, well, then, I should try to gain a couple of pounds.

But I couldn't do it, I couldn't gain weight. I was too afraid of changing the routine, relaxing the control. Sometimes I had a clear sense of what I should do. *I'll just put on an extra couple of pounds. No one will even be able to tell the difference. Besides, I am a little too thin. . . .* But I couldn't maintain that mind-set. Every time I was near food, my whole body grew tight with fear. *I can't eat. . . . Lettuce, Marianne. Just eat the lettuce and a little potato. . . . No. No, I am not going to eat any potato. Feed the potato to the dog. No one's looking now, just get rid of it.* At the moment of control, the moment of being near food, I couldn't let go of the anorexic thinking. I couldn't change my rules and eat the extra food because the inability to eat wasn't about food. It was about coping with myself and my emotions when I had no other way to do so. Having made that kind of investment in controlling my food, I couldn't give up my diet: my need to diet was more important than my need to lose weight.

My body responded to the denial of food by telling me in every way it could that it needed fuel to survive. My stomach gnawed desperately at emptiness, my dry skin flaked, my face grew soft hairs, my knees folded when I got up as if I would faint. My body was panicking. It's as though it were screaming, *I NEED FOOD! Give me food, give me food NOW because I'm starting to collapse! I can't take this much longer, I won't last much longer.* But my mind answered the hunger of my body with a firm no. *Ignore it. I'm not listening to it, I can't feel it. . . . No, I am not feeling it. Nope, uh-uh. No. NO! I'M NOT EATING!*

I felt a pull between the physical need to eat and the emotional need not to eat. If anything or anyone tilted the balance in that tug-of-war toward the physical need by tempting me with food or forcing me to eat, I became aggressive and nasty. My whole equilibrium was threatened, and I responded as anyone would who is trying to protect herself and her reality: I lashed out.

It was Christmas Day when my mother gave me a Greek cinnamon-honey-nut cookie called *fenikia*. With a stern look, my mother told me to eat the dessert my grandmother had made. I was famished that afternoon, in the literal sense of the word. I had especially starved myself since the middle of November in preparation for the tons of food I would encounter on Thanksgiving and Christmas. Despite this attempt at damage control, I avoided eating on the holidays. No appetizers—well, maybe some carrots and celery—and not much dinner except a salad, some string beans, a small slice of turkey. Everyone else had just eaten turkey, ham, bread, feta cheese, *spanakopeta*, *pastichio*, and other Greek delicacies. While they were feasting, I was smelling the aromas and watching food disappear into people's mouths. I had to flex the muscles in my jaw and gut to stop myself from taking more food and feeling the hunger that was eating my stomach.

And now my mother was sticking a cookie in my face.

I had no choice. The whole family was sitting around the table. As I ate the *fenikia* without tasting it, I stared at my mother, my eyes narrowed and my face hardened in a look of pure hate. "Thank you so very much, Grandma." I spoke slowly, my voice deep and low, my words excessively polite. I was reining myself in, staving off the eruption. "And, Mother, always lovely to be with you on such a lovely and festive holiday. . . . But now I don't feel well. Now I am going to my room." I never withdrew the stare from my mother as I pushed my chair from the table and flicked my napkin onto the plate. I exited the dining room and pounded up the stairs. Each slam of my foot released a different emotion—BOOM, anger that I'd been forced to eat the *fenikia*; BOOM, hatred at my mother for making me eat the *fenikia*; BOOM, sadness at having been so mean to my mother and grandmother; BOOM, panic at the extent of my nastiness; BOOM, fear that I'd gained weight from the *fenikia*; BOOM, unhappiness at all of me.

The tension at home wasn't limited to holidays. Since I couldn't listen to the hunger each night at dinner, I felt threatened, caged, controlled by the food that surrounded me. I was forced to smell the food, feel the hunger, want the food, sense the fear that I might lose control over what I ate. One of the ways to stop my hunger was to become nasty—to turn my negative energy and emotion outward.

I stalked my mother in the kitchen when she made dinner, looking with hawkeyes as she poured olive oil into a pan. Ironically, the amount of olive oil she used didn't really matter since I never ate more than a couple of bites of chicken anyway. But that didn't stop the rage from gradually growing inside me: *She's using olive oil. She's trying to make me fat. Goddamn her! That bitch is trying to make me fat!* My eyes narrowed to slits, my mouth tightened to a hard thin line, my jaw clenched until I could hear a ringing in my ears. All this rage and mistrust directed at my mother, and she was completely unaware. She was just making dinner while my mind was churning so hard I felt as if I could scream, hit her, hurt her, hurt me.

Throughout dinner, I calculated, schemed, tried to clear my plate without eating any food. I prepared for the meal by putting several napkins on my lap when I sat down to eat. After spooning some food into my mouth, I wiped my lips with a napkin and spit out the food. I then chewed air and pretended to swallow. The second napkin was positioned on my lap to receive the food I dished into it directly from my plate. *Can she see if I put this chunk of food into my lap now? . . . Shit, I've got to get the dog away from my lap or she'll give me away. . . . What does that look in Mom's eyes mean? Does she know? Did she see?* I was afraid of getting caught—afraid that my mother would take away my anorexia.

I wrapped the first two food-filled napkins into the third napkin so I could make an easy-to-throw-away package of chewed and uneaten food. The fourth napkin remained clean throughout dinner. At the end of the meal, I made an obvious gesture of wiping my mouth and thrusting the empty napkin triumphantly on the table. The purpose of this gesture was to mess with my mother's mind: she may have *thought* she saw me put food in my lap, but if I had done so, what was the explanation for the clean napkin I had just spread on the table? How could anything be wrong?

It wasn't only at dinnertime that my mother and I felt the presence of anorexia in the house. We were both aware of the eating disorder, and aware that we weren't addressing it. We couldn't talk calmly anymore. Every conversation was charged with anger—an anger that let us express the confusion, self-hate, and sadness that was building in each of us. Instead of letting ourselves feel and work through our emotions, we screamed them into submission. Every day we yelled at each other, but we never once said the words "anorexia" or "anxiety attack." We didn't know how to talk about those things. My mother was too panicked and guilt-ridden to learn about eating disorders and talk with me calmly. I was too desperate and reliant on my eating disorder to talk about it and to stop using my mother as an emotional punching bag.

My brother and father weren't active in my emotional life anymore. My brother became a godlike figure: I looked up to him from afar, but he wasn't real for me. We didn't talk honestly about the substance of our lives. As for my father, he was the "activities man." We went to ball games, played tennis, went sailing. When we spent time in these activities, we had fun and felt close. But my father never became involved in the deep issues I struggled with. He never talked with me about them, and he was never the object of the anger I needed to release. He understood what was happening—he started grinding his teeth at night when I was fifteen—but he didn't openly deal with my eating disorder or emotions. That left my mother alone to engage me emotionally.

"What are you *doing?*" Without knocking, my mother had blasted open the door to my room and caught me exercising on my wood floor. "Why are you *doing* this? Why are you getting so thin? Why are you throwing away your food? You look awful! Do you know what you look like? You're too thin! Do you hear me? You're TOO THIN!"

"Get out! You can't come into my room without knocking! Get out!" We started to push each other, hit each other, pierce each other's skin. We were both desperate to get what we wanted: I wanted to keep exercising and to avoid facing my problem; my mother wanted to stop her daughter from hurting herself, to help her daughter be happy, and to assuage her own guilt that she was somehow responsible for my problems.

My mother's threats and angry confrontations didn't work as she intended. They trapped me, increasing my sense of isolation and fear of talking about this thing that had overtaken my life. My parents didn't realize that I needed a calm, loving discussion instead of hysteria and threats to put a stop to my diet.

At one point my mother told me I couldn't go on a school-sponsored trip to the Soviet Union unless I gained some weight. "Mom, how can you say that! George got to go when he was a sophomore! How can you make me stay home?" "Marianne, just gain the weight and you can go." "Bitch," I said as I stared into her eyes. Then I stormed up to my room and vexed about how I could go on the trip without gaining weight.

Three weeks later, I stood on a scale wearing a robe as my mother looked at the needle. "One hundred and eight. I'm fine. Excuse me, I have to pack now, *Mother*." "Oh, okay, good." She was a bit stunned. She didn't expect me to have gained weight. I went to my room and shut the door. I stood motionless and listened hard. When I heard my mother go downstairs, I quickly removed the eight-pound ankle weights I had strapped around my thighs. They had done their job well.

After about a year of anorexia, my mother took me to an obstetrician/gynecologist's office because I had stopped getting my period. Several pregnant women waited in the lobby. *God, how do you control what you eat when you're pregnant? You have to drink milk and stuff.* We waited in the lobby for over an hour. I was the youngest person there. I felt like the women were all looking at me. *No, I'm not pregnant. . . . Do I look pregnant?* They were probably wondering what was wrong with me, the skinny kid whose arms were crossed tight on her chest, whose eyes were hard on her pale face. I didn't want to be there. I didn't want some doctor poking at me.

But she did poke at me, take blood samples, do an internal exam. She didn't explain what she was doing or why she was doing it. She didn't explain that her tools would be so cold inside me. *Damnit. What is she doing to me? Shit, she's touching me with that thing. I can't hold it in me, it hurts. Take it out of me! Get it out of me!* She examined me for less than ten minutes. Then I took off the paper robe, put on my clothes, and went into a little room. And waited.

After another twenty minutes, she came back in. There was nothing wrong, she said, although she would know for sure once the lab results came back. Probably just adolescent irregularity. When I stood up to leave, I felt the familiar nauseating head rush: fuzzy splotches bounced in my vision, a sense of imbalance disoriented my movement, and I wanted to vomit even though I hadn't eaten any food. The head rushes and constant light-headedness were my body's unheeded warnings to stop starving myself.

"Doctor, she's been losing a lot of weight lately." We were practically out the office door when my mother spoke. The doctor paused from writing on her chart. She looked up at me and slid her glasses down her nose. "You know, Marianne, you can eat an ice cream cone if you want. Don't worry about it, you can afford it."

Out we went.

As soon as we were in the car, my mother started with me. "See, Marianne. Let's go get an ice cream cone."

Silence.

"Marianne, Marianne, she *said* you should have an ice cream cone."

"Mom, nothing's wrong with me. The doctor said so. And I do *not* want any *ice cream*. I want to go home. I have homework to do." Work and diet. My island of safety.

# F O U R

■

# From Anorexia to Bulimia

I GOT to my room, panting from fear and excitement. I sat on the wood floor, back curved over my food, body tense in anticipation of the bagel with strawberry jam.

That afternoon I had seen my mother eat a bagel. I had watched her tasting it, crunching it, sucking the crumbs from her fingers. An hour after dinner, during which I successfully threw away most of my food as usual, I walked into the kitchen breathing deep and fast. Looking around me, making sure no one could see me, I slowly took a bagel out of the bread box, covered it with jam, and wrapped it lightly in a paper napkin. I walked rapidly up the stairs, trying to get to my room before anyone saw my napkin-wrapped package, trying to get to my private space so I could eat.

When I was done eating, I went to the bathroom to brush my teeth, to rid myself of the taste of the crime.

"Marianne, *get* over here!" My mother was standing in my

room, pointing to the wood floor. "What's this? What's going on?" I said nothing. "Are you bleeding? What are you doing, Marianne?"

"It's *jelly*, okay! It's not blood, it's jelly! I ate a *bagel* with some *jelly!*" Although the yelling was directed at my mother, the hate was directed at me. This was the first time I had broken my diet and eaten food in secret. I hated myself for having eaten, for having lost control. Along with the hate, I felt confusion, embarrassment, fear, and failure. The screaming quickly tackled those other emotions. It stopped me from feeling anything but rage. Rage was easier for me to handle.

I watched the tension in my mother's face recede as her fearful energy got severed from its source. "Oh. Okay. . . . I'm going downstairs to watch the end of the news with Dad. . . . Um, that jam is good, isn't it? . . . Okay, I'm going downstairs now. . . ." The last two years had trained my mother to be afraid of my emaciation, to watch me put my dinner in the trash can, to see me exercise my little limbs. I was down to about 80 pounds, and she was scared for my health. So when she saw a red splotch on the floor, she logically thought it was blood. Upon realizing the red splotch was jam, she didn't know how to react. We had become used to a reality in which I didn't eat voluntarily. Now reality was shifting, and neither of us knew what that meant.

After another week of anorexic behavior, I had a second episode of uncontrolled eating. Once again, an hour after a family dinner during which I threw away most of my food, I started feeling the need to eat. I quietly walked into the kitchen, looked at the closed freezer, and visualized the ice cream carton resting inside it. I was pulled toward the food, a willing victim of the desire to grab it, feel it, put it in my mouth, eat it.

My mouth embraced the mound of ice cream on the cold spoon. That first taste was both delicate and violent—delicate in the sensual pleasure of tasting; violent in the declaration contained within the act of eating, the declaration that I was free from all outside expectations of how I should look, how I should act, who I should be. After all this dieting, all this lost weight, I still wasn't happy. My weight loss hadn't transformed my social life, my hate, my confusion. By eating, I was saying that I wouldn't play by the same restrictive rules when I knew I couldn't win the game, when I knew I couldn't get the happiness that thinness had promised. By eating, I was saying: "Fuck this, fuck you, fuck everything, I won't do it anymore."

When the cup of ice cream was empty, the energy that had tickled my skin sank back into my body. I breathed deeply a few times, eyes closed, muscles relaxed, until . . . Panic. *What's happening to me? Why am I eating? Why can't I control it? I used to control it, why can't I control it?* My thoughts were fast—calorie calculations, damage assessments, plans to undo the damage, fears I couldn't undo the damage, further calorie calculations, etc. I huddled on the wood floor of my room, arms sealing my knees to my chest, and rocked back and forth. I felt desperate to hold on to my evaporating control over my food, my body, myself. That's when I knew the bingeing didn't free me, when I knew the only thing I fucked by bingeing was myself.

The slide from anorexia to bulimia was natural: both disorders served to soothe me and to allow me to deal with myself in my world, and both used food/body manipulation as the basis for doing so. When I was sixteen, I gravitated toward food physically and emotionally. Physically, my body could no longer survive without nourishment. I could no longer maintain my anorexia, not because I lacked the willpower to diet, but because I retained the physical instinct to survive. Emotionally, I wanted to eat, because this self-denial of food hadn't given me the happiness and confidence I thought it would.

But when I began to feed myself, I couldn't eat in moderation. Since I hadn't dealt with the underlying emotional causes of my anorexia, I still needed a coping mechanism. And since I was still in an anorexic headspace that said eating was evil, I believed that I was pathetic for eating one piece of bread. So when I ate a piece of bread, I told myself that I might as well eat a whole loaf of bread, and I might as well eat that loaf with jam and honey. For that matter, I might as well eat ice cream, too, and cheese and muffins and all those other things I hadn't let myself eat for two years. At the time, I didn't know that I was essentially telling myself, "I might as well switch my coping mechanism from anorexia to bulimia."

Over the next eight years, my eating behavior followed the same stubborn pattern. First, my body and spirit screamed that they wanted food. Second, when I fed myself, the eating was emotionally charged with guilt and risk and self-hate. That charge came from my belief that I wasn't supposed to eat; that there was no pleasurable, healthy, or safe way to eat bread or cake; that I had to choose between obesity and thinness. And that charge was often violent, even sexual, in its intensity: I needed and desired to eat with all of my body and spirit, and I would take any food I could get, regardless of the consequences. Third, when the food was gone, the guilt and hate emerged: I've failed at maintaining my diet; I've broken the pattern; one cookie is as bad as one box of cookies is as bad as two boxes of cookies and ice cream and granola and chocolate and muffins and brownies and . . . Fourth, when I felt as if my bloated body was suffocating my spirit, I purged myself of food by starving myself for the next few days or by exercising heavily or, eventually, by throwing up. Fifth, after I purged my body of food, I felt deprived again, both physically and emotionally. Even though I told myself that I would never binge again, I began needing food. And that's when my body and spirit would scream that they wanted food. And that's when step five became step one and the cycle started over again.

This cycle established itself quickly, but the behaviors associated with each step developed slowly and jerkily. In the first stage, I would eat anorexically when in public but would then secretly eat four pieces of bread or three apples, etc., after the last meal of the day. In the second stage, I would ransack the house for any bit of food for a few days and then eat anorexically for a few days. In the third stage, the ransacking of the house would continue in conjunction with a new behavior: buying food in stores in order to have concentrated periods of massive eating. Once again, this behavior was followed by a period of anorexic eating. In the fourth stage, I would actively binge on large amounts of food in a short time and immediately purge that food by vomiting. I moved from stage one to stage two within six months, and began stage three after another sixteen months. Half a year after that, I began to stick my finger down my throat and vomit my food.

Throughout all these stages—even as the bingeing got bigger and the periods of anorexic eating got shorter—I told myself that the bingeing Marianne wasn't the real me. The bingeing Marianne was the "bad" Marianne. After I binged, the "real" Marianne, the one who was thin and in control, would come back and diet. In this way, I was able to deny that I was becoming bulimic.

UP AND DOWN, bingeing or starving, all or none. I stayed with the "none" for a day, four days, four weeks—as long as my body and spirit could take it. Then I went back to the "all" of bingeing. All or none, all or none. Bingeing one day, starving the next: it felt as if someone were flicking a switch inside me—on and off, on and off, on and off.

As I alternated between these two extremes, I would gain seven pounds, lose five, gain four, lose two. Three months after I ate that first bagel with jam, when I went to my friend Laura's house on the Fourth of July, I weighed a little over 100 pounds. Although I was eating extra pieces of bread and sneaking food when no one could see, I still wasn't eating very much compared with nonanorexic people. But I was gaining weight, and I was losing control.

Laura, whose father was a New York Jets coach at the time, was a competitive swimmer with broad football-player shoulders, a small waist, a quick mind, and a ready, wide smile. Despite all the power in Laura's body, she admired stick-thin people. I had been friends with Laura for a couple of years.

That night Laura's older sister was having a party with some of her college friends. About eight of us were playing Trivial Pursuit. If someone got the answer wrong, he or she had to take a chug of beer. Here I was, socially inept Marianne, playing drinking games with college men! Wow! It was exciting! I mean, they *joked* with me! And I was witty right back! At times like that night, I recognized that my weight gain was positive. I felt my body growing in strength, and I saw my shape swelling from that of a child to that of a woman. I didn't want to go back to weighing 80 pounds. But I did want to go back to the time when I wasn't so desperate to eat.

"That guy's looking at you," Laura whispered to me. I looked at her with big eyes, half in disbelief, half in fear. She took a sip of beer, leaned into me, and kept whispering. "I was talking to Jeff before, and he said all the Cornell guys are sick of college women. Jeff said the women in college all get fat. They want thin girls."

I nodded my head, as if I understood. My face flushed pink as I thought, *But I'm gaining weight! I can't keep it. . . . I'm gonna get fat. You think I look good now, but wait a couple of days, you'll see me get gross! You and everyone else will see me get fat! . . . I'm a disgusting pig, you don't even know it now, but I am, you'll see it soon. You'll see I'm a pig!* I stopped listening to Laura for a few seconds, gathered my thoughts, and decided on a plan of action: *Okay, Marianne. Go on a diet tomorrow, Marianne. You can stay thin. . . . Just go on a diet. You don't have to lose any more weight. Just go on a diet to stay right here, stay right at this weight. . . .*

". . . at you."

"What? I didn't hear you." In my strategizing, I had missed Laura's comment.

"I said that's why that guy is looking at you. Because you're not fat like all the other girls here."

*Be thin. . . . Stay thin. . . . Get control.* Despite the fear, despite the plans to lose weight, I needed to binge, and the bingeing grew worse.

I was calculating the number of hours I had to wait for my parents to go to bed so I could get food from the kitchen. It was 8 P.M.

*Shit! She's having coffee! Oh no, no, no, Mom, don't have so much coffee! . . . Damn. . . . Okay, it's okay. By ten o'clock she'll be upstairs. Okay, so two hours. Two more hours. Then she'll go upstairs and I can eat.* Ten o'clock came. My mother was still downstairs. *Damnit. Get upstairs. GO TO BED! GET UPSTAIRS!* I was starting to panic. I felt anger toward my mother. I needed to eat food and she wouldn't let me have it. By staying awake, she was preventing me from meeting my needs.

My mother went to bed at 10:30. I had been tired, but when she left, my energy level rose. I could eat now. I waited for the sound of my parents shutting their bedroom door. I stepped into the bathroom and flushed the toilet so the sound of water moving through the pipes would temporarily cover the sounds of my search for food. I crept into the kitchen, tiptoed to the refrigerator, and opened the door slowly so the jars didn't clang together. *Yes! Some leftover potato stew . . . and some cheese. . . .* I ate, fast, greedy. *That's it. No more.* Five minutes passed. Six minutes. Up from the couch, groping through the cabinets, searching for cookies or peanuts or crackers or chocolate.

Even though I wasn't cold, I wrapped myself in a maroon mohair blanket on the couch before starting to eat the crackers I had found. The folds of the blanket let me hide the food in case my mother came downstairs. I knew the sound of her moving in the house. A creak told me which room she was in, whether she was moving closer to me, how many seconds I had to hide the food. If I heard her approach, I would hide the food in the blanket and hold a book over my face until I finished chewing.

Over the next year, the periods between uncontrolled eating got shorter, the amount I ate got larger, and the things I did to get food became more desperate. My brother was at Princeton now; the house felt hollow, and the opportunities to eat grew. "Mom, I'll clean the dishes." "Okay, thanks." She began clearing the table. "Mom, get out of the kitchen! I said I would do the dishes!" "Oh, I was just helping, I . . . ." "Let me do them. If you don't want me to do them, fine, but I said I would do them." My voice was hard. I needed to be alone in the kitchen. I needed to be alone so I could eat.

That day I had followed my new pattern: I hadn't eaten anything since breakfast, when I had a bowl of cereal, and I was starving by dinner—starving for food, and for the opportunity to eat in secret. When my mother left the kitchen, I looked around to gauge the locations of everyone else in the house. I grabbed the leftover spaghetti and meat sauce in my right hand and clumped it into my mouth. Ringing filled my ears. Excited, nervous, plotting energy filled my body. Eat what's left on Mom's plate, eat what's left in the pot. Sauce under my fingernails, sauce on my face. Wipe off the sauce, breathe fast, grab the bread, eat it in the bathroom sitting on the toilet.

That night we had enough leftovers for me to eat. But on some nights I had to search for food in the garbage or take scraps out of the dog's bowl. Whatever I could get, whatever I could find.

A weekend later that month, I was looking for my brother's copy of the play *Waiting for Godot*. As I took it off the shelf, I saw a little picture of butter cookies—the kind that dance along the outside of a cookie tin. Slowly, deliberately, I pulled out the tin and opened the top. My mother's oatmeal raisin cookies were smooshed inside. I breathed long and slow to taste the smell.

My mother had hidden food from me before. Cookies, Entenmann's cakes, peanut butter, bread were all camouflaged around the house. I found food folded in sweaters in my mother's closet, perched on the rims of crystal wineglasses in the dining room cabinet, and now here, on my brother's bookcase behind Sartre, Mann, and Camus.

When I saw those oatmeal raisin cookies, my emotions left me. Energy zipped along my hands, my back, my cheeks. Then the energy became focused, settling on the target. Eating would calm me down. Eating would take away emotion.

I ate two cookies. *Good. . . . Oh, they taste so sweet!* I focused on the sweetness, the chewiness in my mouth, the softness of the raisins. *Good. They're good. . . . Another one. I'll just get two more. . . . These are so good. A few more, just a few more.* Five cookies, eight, twelve, thirteen. My mouth was dry, the cookies tasted like sawdust. But I kept eating. *Two more, that's it. Okay, move the cookies around the tin so Mom can't tell so many are gone. . . .*

I replaced the tin box behind the books. The energy of the binge was evaporating and the emotions were returning: confusion, self-hate, fear, embarrassment. *You're pathetic, Marianne! You drive your own mother to sneak around the house hiding food! You're disgusting, you piece of shit! You out-of-control piece of shit! . . . What will Mom do when she finds the cookies gone? . . . Maybe she won't be able to tell. . . . Marianne, get real, of course she can tell. Half of them are gone! . . . Will she tell Dad? . . . Damnit, what a bitch for hiding the cookies from me! How could Mom do that to me! Bitch!* I wanted to scream those words so they would no longer echo in my shaking body.

With the food disappearing, the sound of the refrigerator opening each night, and the weight filling out my body, I couldn't keep the "secret" from my family. My mother was the primary person who actively shared my struggle, just as she was when I was anorexic. We never talked about the fears and sadness we both felt, the way the eating disorder and its underlying causes created so much hurt within both of us. Usually we argued over inherently meaningless issues: my mother looked at me the wrong way, I spoke in a tone of voice my mother didn't like, my mother asked me too many questions. Only twice did we argue about food.

"I thought we had another loaf of bread. I wonder what happened to that bread, Marianne. Someone must've eaten it, right, Marianne?" She was looking me in the eye, speaking slowly and coolly. Her chilly tone and staring eyes said: *I know what you did. I know you ate the bread.*

Embarrassment started in my gut and slid through my body; my hands tingled and went numb. I felt cornered. And like all animals who feel cornered, I charged. "I guess so, Mom. But you would know, wouldn't you, since you don't have a job and just sit around the house all day. Right, Mom?" My body stood rigidly, muscles tense, bread anchored inside me. My mother and I were stuck, unable to feel and deal with our emotions.

The second argument was more explosive. The family was on vacation in the Hamptons on the east end of Long Island, where Manhattanites summer. East Hampton is like my hometown, Garden City, except everyone wears bathing suits. I had been bingeing every day of the vacation—Fig Newtons, bagels, muffins, lasagna. My mother knew I had been eating a lot, she was watching me gain weight, she was seeing leftovers disappear. So she looked in my purse, where I had stuffed two donuts to be eaten later.

"Get out of my bag!" I shrieked at her.

"What are you doing, Marianne! You've got two donuts in there! What are you doing! Are you hungry? Yes, you're hungry? Then *eat* a dozen donuts, *eat* bread, *eat* boxes of cereal! Are you hungry, Marianne? Then EAT!" Her eyes were wild.

I was caught, and I was humiliated. "What are you *doing, bitch*! You're such a bitch! How could you look in my bag?! That's *my* bag!"

"Don't call me a bitch! Do you want us to help you through college? If you do, you start treating me with *respect*. Or that's it, you're out of here."

"*Fuck you.*" That did it. I could see the froth at the side of her mouth. She grabbed my hair, yanking my head back and forth. I dug my nails into her skin. We were so unhappy. But we didn't feel unhappiness at that moment. All we felt was hysteria. Angry hysteria.

That afternoon was the one time my father became involved. Usually, when he came home from a long workday and was forced to hear the yelling between his wife and his daughter, he would listen until he couldn't ignore it anymore. Then he would yell. "Frances, Marianne, stop it! Go to your rooms! I don't want to hear this anymore! This is bullshit! You're yelling at each other over nothing!" A husband telling his own wife to go to her room—it was an odd situation. But that afternoon in East Hampton was different. He got involved. Maybe because he was in the middle of a two-week vacation and could focus on his family more than usual, maybe because relatives were in the house to witness the screaming—I'm not sure why he got involved, but he did. He sat on the bed as my mother stood in one corner of the room and I in the other. He asked me what I was feeling, he asked my mother why she had looked in my bag, he asked me why I had bought the food, he asked my mother if she could give me some space, he asked both of us if we could apologize. We did, and the fighting subsided for the moment. I remember feeling surprised and relieved that my father had intervened. He grounded my mother and me that afternoon. But that was the only time. And even that day, none of us mentioned the words "bulimia" or "eating disorder."

Part of me felt lucky that my parents didn't calmly discuss bulimia with me. Discussing it would have removed some of its power: part of the release associated with bulimia is the secretiveness—turning from other people and shutting off emotions, being deviant when normalcy means following rules and expectations, being in your own world where no one can touch you. I needed that release. I didn't want anyone to diminish it or take it away. But at the same time, I was hurting and needed help.

When my brother came home on vacations from Princeton, he saw that I was gaining weight. He thought the outcome was good—he was glad I wasn't sickly thin. But the process—the bingeing and the anger that came with it—distressed him. My brother didn't talk about my eating disorder with me, not when he came downstairs and caught me eating a whole cake, not when I finished off a whole box of his favorite cereal. But one day the yelling between my mother and me pushed my brother too far. "Marianne, you're pissed at Mom because she hovers over you. Mom, you're pissed at Marianne because she eats in her room. So just leave each other alone! Get out of each other's way! Marianne, you go to your room. Mom, you go to yours. I hate coming home and hearing you guys fight! Screw this, I'm going back to Princeton early. I don't need to deal with this on my vacation. Go on screaming if you want to, I'm leaving." And he slammed the door. And I felt guilty. I was ruining the family.

I COULDN'T EVER get rid of my body. I couldn't ever live outside my skin. My body became a billboard announcing to everyone that I was a pathetic, deviant failure. It became proof of my disgusting behavior, my lack of control, my abnormality.

My body became the battleground where I played out my emotions. *Look at you, Marianne. Look at that gut. Disgusting. It blobs like cottage cheese.* I was naked in front of my mirror. *Look at these arms. My thighs used to be that big! Disgusting, Marianne. . . . Do some push-ups, Marianne, get your arms small again. This is disgusting!* I looked in the mirror and saw flabby arms, fatty hips, a rounded belly. I saw myself piece by piece by piece. I didn't see the connections. I didn't see a form composed of curves and straight edges, of soft tissue and strong muscles. I didn't see *me.* My body image reflected my self-image: I hated my body because I hated myself, I doubted my body because I doubted myself, I was angry at my body because I was angry at myself. Hate, doubt, anger. That's what I saw when I looked in the mirror.

I wore long shirts with lots of material to cover my gut. I bought pants and skirts with elastic waistbands to stretch over my alternately expanding and shrinking body. I had "fat" clothes and "thin" clothes—clothes that fit when I was binge-ing and clothes that fit when I was dieting. Each day I started my morning in dread as I tried to find something to wear.

That hatred of myself and my body made me doubt that any guy could ever like me, including Sal, the guy who asked me to the Winter Wonderland dance in December of my junior year. Janice, Sal, Mike, and I were in physics lab together that year. I felt comfortable with our group and our teacher Mr. Maloney, a friendly guy with buckteeth, thick dirty glasses, and a palpable enthusiasm about science. Sal had a gravelly voice and big brown eyes. His intelligence, artwork, and personality weren't mainstream, but they were his, and he knew they were his. He didn't need to run toward some other idea, person, or image to make himself whole.

The night of the dance, I was a mess. *Does this dress look okay? What are we gonna talk about? He doesn't even want to go with me! It's gonna be so awkward! What should I do when we go out to dinner? I can't eat anything, I can't let him see me eat anything. Should I drink, should I pretend I'm drinking? What am I doing? Sal doesn't like me, this is ridiculous.* I radiated nervous energy, creating a shield so that no one, including Sal, could get close to my body or my person.

"Sal, I have to find the Winter Wonderland Queen nominees. I'll be right back, okay?" Before I could hear his response, I dove into the tangle of people. I was thankful to have the responsibility of running the Winter Wonderland contest—a contest in which the students voted on the prettiest senior in the school. I had organized the survey, counted the votes, bought the long-stemmed red roses to go with the long bodies and red lips of the six nominees. At the dance, I spent my time looking around for the six seniors to ensure that they had their roses and weren't too drunk to mount the podium. That task was my excuse to avoid my date, to avoid experiencing the moment of being at the dance in a black velvet dress with a date who wanted to be with me. Sal and I ended the night awkwardly, without a kiss, and I felt uncomfortable for the rest of the year in physics.

A LITTLE OVER a year after I went from anorexia to bulimia, I binged on cereal, bread, peanuts, and a banana, not yet totally ripe, a little too firm. I tried to sleep. It was hot. I was sweating, restless in my bed. The food seemed to have settled high in my chest. I burped and tasted acid in my mouth. I started pacing the room. My stomach hurt so much; it was distended, stretching my skin thin over my belly. I whimpered. Finally, as I paced, I bent over and threw up on my bedroom floor, without using my finger as I would in the future. My body rejected the food that clogged it. Again I threw up. And then I could breathe.

My mother knew about what happened that August night. A few days later, she finally took action. "Marianne, why don't you . . . I got the number of a place, right near here, it's the Diet Center, and . . . you've been so sad lately, and maybe this can help." My mother told me she would accompany me to the first meeting if I wanted her to; she said she would pay for it. Determined to help me, she decided that the solution to my sadness and anger and eating was the Diet Center. As if all my problems would disappear if I could just get control of my weight. As if the binges were the root of my emotions, not the other way around.

At first I was embarrassed that my mother had suggested the Diet Center. But then I decided that she was right: I was sad, and here she was telling me calmly, reassuringly that she had the name and number of someone who could help, that many good people went there, that going didn't mean something was wrong with me. At the time, I didn't realize that diet programs provide only a temporary "fix" because they don't address the deeper reasons people use food—they don't help people learn how to deal with themselves in their world in a healthy way.

I felt hot as I filled out the questionnaire. *How much do you weigh?* . . . 160 pounds. *Why do you want to lose weight?* . . . To look better. *Have you ever been anorexic or bulimic?* . . . No.

"Hi." My diet counselor was smiling. She seemed nice. "We're gonna take a 'before' picture now to put in your file, and after you lose weight, we'll take an 'after' picture and you'll be able to see the difference." Snap. I was wearing orange elastic-waistband shorts and a loose black top. A drop of sweat formed on my back as my counselor measured the size of my calf, thigh, hips, waist, upper arm, chest.

The counselor was sitting behind the desk, analyzing the paperwork. "Your goal weight should be 116 pounds," she said, nodding her head in reassurance. "You can go over 116, but that should be your goal. Okay! This'll be fun!"

I was giddy when I left the Diet Center that first day. I was on the road back to thinness and happiness, I thought. I had a plan and rules; I had food charts, exercise charts, weight charts, all to plot my progress. *This is it, Mare. I can be thin again! Maybe I can lose ten pounds before school starts. . . . Ten pounds, okay, I can do that!*

In the next few months, I followed the charts and I lost the weight. I felt good about my body. I went for walks, exercised, bought new clothes. Each Sunday I plotted exactly what I would eat for the next seven days. I plotted when and how much I would exercise. I locked my head back into an anorexic mind-set. I got deeper into the "all or none" headspace.

"Two more pounds this week, Marianne! Just thirty pounds to go!" I had to prove to my counselor what a good dieter I was; I had to pass the test each week as I stood on the scale and my counselor nudged the weights downward. "One and three quarters pounds this week!" "You're my best dieter, Marianne!" I lost fifty pounds in three months. I got compliments from classmates, teachers, my diet counselor. I felt so successful, so high, when they commented on my weight loss. "How'd you do that?" some girls would ask, and I sensed wonderment and awe in their voices. "Jeez, how much weight have you lost, Marianne?" "Keep it up, Marianne." "Good for you, Marianne." I'd done it—I was in control again, and it showed.

After losing so much weight and feeling attractive in my stylish new clothes, I broke. I ate a piece of bread with cheese—both foods that were not allowed on the Diet Center diet, and that were not allowed with my all-or-none mind-set. As I ate that bread and cheese, I knew I would keep on eating, keep on chewing, keep on taking, until my stomach became a bloated bulge. "None" clicked back to "all": I'd broken the spell, I'd eaten, I'd failed, and since I'd failed, I might as well feed my pathetic self all the food it wanted. The next day, like an omen of the upcoming years of purging, I threw up as a result of a migraine headache. The migraine, plus the pain and purging related to it, was a release—a purging of the pressure to keep to my diet.

I was now afraid of my Diet Center counselor. "Mom, please call them, I don't want to go anymore. Please! I can't go anymore!" Panic filled my words and throat. What would my counselor think? She'd praised me when I'd lost all that weight; what would she think of me now? *She'll hate me now. I'm pathetic. I'm gaining all the weight back!* They had already put my "before and after" photographs on their Wall of Success. I couldn't go back now that I was a failure.

I could avoid the counselors, but I couldn't avoid all the people who had complimented me, all my peers and relatives who had seen me get skinny. I felt people were watching me, watching my waistband stretch. I felt I was ballooning up, bursting out in front of people. Each day getting fatter and fatter and fatter. *They're laughing. Why are they laughing?* I had just walked into French class. Maura and Margaret—two tall, popular women—were sharing a secret. *They're talking about me. I must be getting so fat. Oh my God, these pants are disgusting. They're laughing at my pants, at these fucking elastic-waistband pants!* It never occurred to me that Maura and Margaret had lots of things to discuss other than my weight.

But my fear of a nasty peer reaction to my weight gain was in part justified. "Marianne is fat." Heat filled my gut and spread to my cheeks. "Marianne is fat." It was written in pen on a desk in the library—my favorite desk, where I worked for an hour each afternoon. I looked around. *Who wrote this? What bitch wrote this? . . . Marianne, you are fat, and here someone has written it down for you so you can see it every day. Every fucking day.* That note reflected the character of Garden City. Many kids in that wealthy community, including me, had all the material things they wanted. Many kids felt they were always entitled to what they had—that the pleasures of life came without cost, without any responsibility on their part. In addition, in this homogeneous town, we weren't among different kinds of people whose values, looks, rituals, and traditions varied. The community therefore lacked an acceptance of difference and the compassion for others that can come with diversity. The combination of overabundance and sameness hurt the adolescent community of Garden City. Some parents gave their kids responsibilities and emphasized the virtues of diversity, acceptance, openness, and challenge. But some didn't. And I think that's why someone felt she or he could write "Marianne is fat," and why no one erased it for weeks.

A month after I broke my Diet Center diet—the winter of my senior year—I started a new pattern of full-out binges: going from store to store to buy food, planning binges days in advance. When I binged, I was in a different reality. The bingeing let me enter a world where there were no rules, no expectations—not of getting an A or doing well on the AP exams or fitting in at parties. I didn't have to be a perfect girl when I was in this world. I could be bad. I could ignore the rules, and no one would judge me. I stayed in this world while planning and executing a binge. But I returned to the other world—the "real" world—when the food was gone. Then the rules returned, the pressures returned, and the judgments returned. All of which led me to binge again.

I planned to binge when my parents had a social engagement on the weekends. *Three full hours alone. . . .* Enough to buy food and eat it. *Only eight more days, Marianne, and they'll be gone for three full hours. . . .* When I couldn't be alone in the house, I drove around town eating food in my mother's white Volvo. One typical day I bought a box of cookies and two muffins at two different stores, then I went to crown my binge with frozen yogurt. I got nervous as I walked into the frozen yogurt shop and came face-to-face with someone who knew I was about to eat.

"Hi. Um, I'll have, um, I guess, let's see, uh . . . vanilla, in a cup. . . ." It was hard for me to make a decision because thoughts zipped in and out of my head, confusing me. *Okay, so okay, so I'm buying frozen yogurt. . . . Okay, it's okay, Marianne. Just don't have yogurt or cookies or muffins after today. No more. . . . But I . . . But the guy in the store will see me buy the yogurt. He'll know I'm pigging out and . . . He'll know! . . . Damnit, Marianne, calm down! Calm yourself! Marianne, the guy works in a frozen yogurt shop. . . . He serves people yogurt all day. He doesn't care that you're getting yogurt. He doesn't care. . . .* "Those, um, those toppings look great. . . . I'll, um, maybe I'll get one. . . . Okay, I'll be really bad and get the, um, the chocolate crunch topping. . . . I really shouldn't, but I've had a tough day, so, um, I'll do it. . . ." The last comment was a justification for eating the topping, just as my father always justified eating a full meal. I was letting the yogurt scooper know I didn't normally do this sort of thing: I had a complete understanding of the fact that I was doing a bad thing, that I shouldn't be eating this food, and that eating it was a onetime exception. I was thereby short-circuiting any criticism he might have of me.

I was smiling, trying to look completely comfortable with myself so I could convince the yogurt scooper that I didn't have any problem whatsoever with buying frozen yogurt. If I smiled, I could diffuse any suspicion that I might be bingeing. *I'm just some person buying frozen yogurt, no big deal. There's no reason to suspect me of bingeing. None. I'm cool, I'm smiling. He has no reason to suspect me. Keep smiling. Get the yogurt and get out of the store. . . . Come on, put more topping on, damnit, I want the topping! Okay, it's okay. Keep smiling.*

"Why shouldn't you have a topping?" He was looking at me as he added luscious chocolate crunchies to my yogurt.

"Huh? . . ." His question seemed so strange. *Why shouldn't I? It's frozen yogurt! It's a dessert! And I'm putting chocolate on it! I just . . . I mean, I just can't. . . . It's not something that I . . . it's fat!* "Well, I'm just, I'm on a diet."

"Oh. . . . Why?"

I was too perplexed to realize he was flirting with me. *Why?*

*Why am I on a diet? Just because. Because that's just the way it is. I should always be on a diet. That's just the way I should eat.* "Just, you know, to keep in shape. You know. . . ." I don't think he knew. And I don't think I knew why I needed my eating habits, either. I took the yogurt and moved toward the door, fast. "Thanks. Bye."

I drove to the parking lot of the Garden City library and ate six cookies from the box. I checked my face in the rearview mirror to make sure I didn't have chocolate crumbs in my teeth, and I walked into the library. After reading in a cubicle for a while, cautiously, slowly, I gathered up my bag and walked to the bathroom. I locked myself in the single stall and ate the remaining cookies and melting frozen yogurt. *Please, please, no one knock. . . . Oh, this is good. . . . Am I taking too long in here? . . . The cookies taste good with this yogurt. . . .* I paused to flush the toilet so no one would get suspicious, then I finished my stash.

The library bathroom seemed like the logical place for me to eat: I needed the food, I wouldn't be bothered in the bathroom, and I was afraid I couldn't smuggle food past my mother and eat it at home. If the point of eating had been to taste and enjoy the food, doing it in the bathroom would have been counterproductive. But since the point was the *idea* of eating—the idea of allowing myself to scoop frozen yogurt into my mouth, allowing myself to buy and consume an entire box of cookies—the bathroom was just fine.

MY FRIENDS COULDN'T know. They couldn't know about the lack of control, the bingeing, the lying. If they knew, they would feel as much disgust toward me as I felt toward myself. Instead of confiding in them, I lied to them: I told them I had been anorexic, that the anorexia had destroyed my metabolism to the point where I currently gained weight even if I barely ate anything. It was an obvious lie. But I repeated it because I didn't trust my friends: I didn't trust them with my fears, my guilt, my rage, my secret. I didn't trust them enough to make myself vulnerable to them. They might betray me. I felt safer alone.

But part of me didn't want to be alone. Part of me wanted to be with people I thought I could trust. I found those people toward the end of my senior year. I was doing the student council thing, going to homerooms giving out election ballots. One homeroom located in a small dark hole in the school consisted of three or four guys who engineered the school assemblies. The room contained some beat-up old couches, wires for recording and lighting, a guitar, some Grateful Dead posters. It was a hideaway. I liked it.

The people in that homeroom, plus their friends, were involved in meetings about changing the school smoking policy. As president of the student council, I took part in the discussion about eliminating the designated smoking area located outside the school. At first, I was in favor of a ban on smoking: smoking is bad for people's health, I had never smoked, and my friends preferred Budweiser to Camel. But there was a contingent of smokers and their friends who came to all the meetings. They wore black clothes or untucked flannel shirts. Some of the girls wore thick black eyeliner—not your typical makeup look in Garden City. They argued persuasively, quietly, for their cause: the existence of the smoking area did not encourage students to smoke, it provided a space for students to smoke who were already doing so. If such an area didn't exist, students would either smoke in the bathrooms or walk off school grounds to smoke during lunchtime.

I hated cigarettes—their smell, their taste, their damaging effects. But the smoking area was more than a place for students to light up cigarettes, it was a gathering place for a certain social group. This group—which included people who smoked and people who didn't—rejected the mainstream values of Garden City High. Instead of trying to adapt to values and situations they didn't like, and instead of feeling alienated from all social situations, they created their own scene with their own values and their own definitions of what it meant to have fun.

A girl in my Latin class was in this group. She and I shared a sense of dissatisfaction with Garden City, but she found satisfaction in her group of friends while I found it only in food. One afternoon, when I bumped into Nathalie at her locker on the way to Latin, she was listening to her Walkman. "Listen to this," she said. "Great song." John Lennon's "Imagine" filled my head. If you haven't heard the song, buy the album, go into a cool, dark room alone, and listen. The song is lonely, like a man standing alone without any defenses saying what he feels in his soul. As I listened in the hallways of Garden City High School, I felt connected to the strength and energy of people who wanted a change, who were unhappy with the state of the world around them.

I was attracted to this energy and these people—the guys in the hideaway homeroom, the smokers' advocates, Nathalie and her musical taste. But even though I was drawn to the group, I couldn't be in it. I couldn't let go of what I thought I was supposed to be, who I thought I was supposed to hang out with. In their dress, words, attitudes, and actions, members of that group questioned traditions and authority, and they embodied experience. I wasn't ready for that. I wasn't ready to feel okay with who I was, to explore who I was, to openly reject my community and the values it proclaimed. I wasn't ready to accept experience, to live life instead of fearing it, to give up control for mystery, to open myself to rejection but also to connection, growth, and laughter.

Instead of exploring with Nathalie and her friends, I looked toward the future, anxiously hoping that it would bring me happiness and free me from bingeing. After all, my problem wasn't me, my problem was my suburban high school, my mother, my community. I held on tight to that belief, in terror that it was wrong.

THE SUMMER AFTER I graduated from high school, I kicked off my new life by studying at the Sorbonne in Paris. For the first two weeks in Paris I suppressed my self-doubt and sadness by immersing myself in the fantasy that I had started a new, binge-free, thin life filled with dating and happiness and wildness. I actually did start a new life when I was in Paris—a more mature, independent, and self-aware life, but one that still included my coping mechanism. I explored museums, traveled to Germany for the Roger Waters/Pink Floyd concert at the fallen Berlin Wall, read *For Whom the Bell Tolls* on the banks of the Seine. I put away my map and wandered.

In the gardens of Fontainebleau, a mansion on the outskirts of Paris, I talked with my friend Christina, a woman in her late twenties who was learning French for her business. That afternoon Christina said simply, "I'm really glad I'm a woman." "What do you mean?" I asked. Her statement represented a new way of thinking for me. "I mean, I'm glad I'm a woman and not a man because we can be more expressive of our emotions, and we can be really delicate and sensual. But at the same time we can be strong and intelligent. I like being a businesswoman, and I like being feminine." I nodded my head slowly. We sat, not speaking for a while, both feeling the beauty of Fontainebleau and the beauty of the afternoon. "I'm gonna go for a walk, Christina. Let's meet back here in an hour." I wanted to wander in my mind, my feelings, and my environment. As I floated through the maze of bushes at the palace, feeling the energy and heat of the sun and wind, I thought about Christina's words. That afternoon I began to develop an awareness of myself as a woman.

As that awareness grew, I became interested in a classmate of mine—a college senior with intelligence and a highly flirtatious manner. I was more attracted by the *idea* of Todd than to Todd himself. I could project onto him my desire to find a man who was unlike the ones who had rejected me in high school. I thought he could make me blissful and keep me thin. After all, I thought, if I had a man, I would have no need for an eating disorder. A man would make me happy. Besides, I would *have* to stop bingeing then, because we would be fooling around and I would have nowhere to hide.

I have a different view now. I realize that I can't be healed unless I assume responsibility for making changes. No man, no person, can be responsible for changing my eating behavior or my view of myself except me.

After a couple of weeks in Paris, I realized Todd wasn't interested in me. When Todd's rejection killed my fantasy of a new, wild, exciting life, I started bingeing once or twice each day. I stumbled through Paris, going from one patisserie to the next, buying a croissant or pain au chocolat, eating crepes on the street. I walked to burn calories, to find new places to buy food, to avoid thinking about my eating and my unhappiness. *Why am I eating so much? I'm here in Paris, why aren't I happy? . . . Why did I just eat that crepe? That was my third crepe today! And I have two croissants in my bag. Get a grip on yourself. Damnit, Marianne. You're pathetic. Pathetic! You come to this romantic city and all you can do is sit alone and eat. None of the guys are attracted to you. You don't fit into your jeans. You're still not fluent in French. You make me sick!*

Then one day I made myself vomit. I came home from a walk and ate a box of European-style chocolate-covered cookies. I was crying as I walked to the sink in my room, where I stuck my finger down my throat for the first time. At first I didn't throw up. But I stopped crying, I stopped thinking about the fact that I was forcing myself to vomit, and I started concentrating on the task. I thought about the angle of my finger in my throat, about using my stomach muscles to help me get rid of the food, about wiggling my finger to trigger the purge. My concentration was successful.

After I vomited, I washed out my mouth with water and crawled back to bed. I told myself that I would be fine, that I would diet tomorrow. I told myself that I would never do it again. But I cried myself to sleep. I knew it was just the beginning.

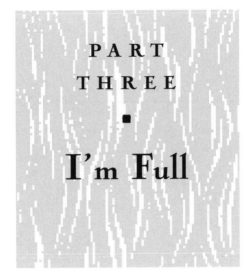

PART
THREE

I'm Full

# FIVE

■

# College Pressures

LILLIAN was one of the first people I met at college. This smart Texas woman had a beautiful round face—white skin, big eyes, bright smile. But her face was the only round thing about her. Her legs were straight rods, her arms gangly, her breasts like a twelve-year-old girl's. Lillian's fragile body could be snapped apart. I wanted to snap her apart because she was too close to me: she was what I was and what I hated— obsessive about food, dishonest about eating; she was what I wanted to be and what I admired—thin, in control. I could spot lots of anorexic women on campus by the way they looked and by their behavior around food. I could spot some bulimic women by their behavior, but there were more than I could see. It's estimated that 10 to 15 percent of students on college campuses have an eating disorder. That percentage shoots up when one includes students with disordered eating or disordered thoughts about food and body.

College is a unique breeding ground for ideas. In my four years as a student at Princeton University, I could feel myself changing, maturing, opening myself to new perspectives. But college is also a unique breeding ground for eating disorders, and I let mine develop into daily binges followed by daily vomiting.

Work pressure at college often leads to eating disorders or disordered eating. During my four years at school, I never had a moment when work pressure didn't throb in my mind: finish one book, start the next; finish one paper, write the next; finish one exam, start the next. Read, write, edit, study, without ever finding peace. In this atmosphere, the easiest way to turn off my mind and get into my body was to binge.

Like many others at college, I never found a safe place where I could release that work pressure. For three years of college, my dorm room wasn't my space, it was the ten-by-twelve-foot area between four walls where I slept. I had one room, crammed with a bed, a computer, books, pictures, clothes, and, for one year, a roommate. I had plenty of places where I could analyze theories of international relations, and plenty of library corners where I could read Kurt Vonnegut. But I had nowhere quiet and private to let my energy settle, to let myself process that energy. As a result, I didn't know what it felt like to relax— relax my muscles, my face, my mind, my self.

Although most of us were feeling stressed and insecure, I let myself believe that everyone else had it together—that I was pathetic compared with my peers on campus. Princeton was brimming with people selected for their range of talents, and the atmosphere was alive with creativity. But the comparisons I created in my mind were deadening me. The people with whom I compared myself were all in my face on this small campus—the thinkers, intellectual innovators, activists, athletes, actors, pianists, socialites—and I didn't know what I was or where I fit in. I just knew I wasn't as good as they were.

Many of my comparisons focused on the body and physical attractiveness. The social and emotional nature of college life is such that there is often pressure to "look good" and stay thin, especially since hundreds or thousands of young people are together in a small space. Each day along the main walkway on campus, my eyes focused on the shadowy figures of women flapping their arms to the *thump-thump* of aerobics music. I would look away from the gym windows toward the walkway, where my eyes focused on tight men, tight women, wearing makeup, being thin. *I must look like that. I must make myself look like that.*

As I floated depressed through Princeton, I longed for the structure my parents had imposed when I lived at home—a structure that at least gave me some degree of security. Each person in college is responsible for her/his independence. Since I wasn't prepared for that responsibility, I took my binge-ing and purging to a new level of intensity. I wasn't the only one unprepared, though: on my hallway alone during freshman year, my neighbor had unprotected sex with various partners, and the guy several doors down got drunk and destructive each weekend.

Despite all the stresses of college life, Princeton gave me the opportunity to redefine myself, to mature. I took that opportunity, but I couldn't do so without holding tight to my coping mechanism in food.

THE SECOND MONTH of school, three sophomores introduced me to Princeton's social center—"the Street." The Street is home to Princeton's nine "eating clubs," which are like coed sororities and fraternities in that they form the hub of the school's social scene, provide bands and lots of cheap beer, and serve meals to club members. Some are "bicker" clubs, meaning people are chosen to join the club after a "rush" process; others are sign-in clubs where a computer randomly selects groups of friends. That night we went to Cottage Club, an elite bicker club—the club where my brother was a member.

We were in the basement, where the beer flowed from kegs and people played cards and talked and flirted. I hated beer with all its calories and intoxication, so no drinking for me. I was too self-conscious to let myself relax, so not much talking or flirting, either. I saw guys wearing jeans and shirts that hugged their muscles. I saw baseball caps adorning smiling faces. I saw women, thin women with little skirts and lots of makeup, curvy women who were charming men or laughing or wearing clothes well. I felt stupid. All over again, I felt like the socially retarded, ugly little high school girl who had nothing to say and who emanated anxious energy. So when someone spilled a large cup of beer on me, I screamed.

"Goddamnit! Watch it! . . . I gotta get out of here. I'm leaving. Excuse me . . . can you move please? . . . Shit, can't you people move!" I pushed through the mingling bodies, past the abstract sounds of words and laughter, and left the club. I was walking down the Street lined with eating clubs and hearty partyers on their way to release the stress of the week. "Marianne!" It was one of the sophomores I'd come with. "What's wrong with you? You can't just storm off like that. That was rude." She was yelling at me. People were looking.

"Katharine, I don't want to talk about it." I started walking fast, face staring at the sidewalk to avoid the eyes I could feel watching me. Katharine was speed-walking right next to me, not letting me get away. "I feel so fat with all those women. I don't like it there. . . . I can't flirt like they all do, I feel so ugly. It's like I can't even control anything anymore! . . . I ate three muffins today, and four bagels and an apple with peanut butter! . . . And I'm bingeing and it's . . . I can't even control myself!" She stopped walking, and I obeyed the command of her action.

"Marianne," she said calmly, her open face and unwavering voice indicating that she was about to say something so simple, so obvious, that it had to be heeded. "Marianne, it's just what you put in here." She was pointing into her mouth. *It's just what I put into my mouth*, she thought. *As easy as that. Just control what I put in my mouth and it'll all be fine. I'll be more social, more fun, more happy. Okay*, I thought. *Okay, she's right, it's just what I put in my mouth. . . . But she's wrong! How could she say that? How could she say I'm feeling all this shit because of food! . . . But maybe she's right. It's just food, Marianne. Damnit, it's just food.* If it were just food, as Katharine said, I wouldn't have spent ten years of my life trying to deal with it.

Since I felt like a worthless person who couldn't contribute anything except in the intellectual realm, I couldn't yet experience by *doing*, as I found out each time I went to the Street. But I started to experience by *observing*. That helped me move to the next stage, where I felt comfortable doing, and it gave me an internal reason to let go of my eating disorder.

I saw the purple flyer on the A floor of Firestone, the main campus library: "Workers needed in the kitchen of Terrace Club to prepare for winter festivities." Terrace Club is an "alternative" eating club where many of Princeton's disaffected find a home. George hated Terrace because he thought it was weird there. I was afraid of Terrace—afraid of its alternative label and its reputation for licentiousness and hedonism. But I immediately called after seeing that purple flyer. I wanted the money. And I wanted a chance to see what licentiousness and hedonism were like.

Terrace Club was dark. The predominant colors were black and blood red. A din of smoke clung to the ceiling and curtains. The chef, Barton, was more like an inspiration than a cook. Thanks to Barton's energy, the club radiated magic and life, which let a lot of Princetonians lose their problems for a while. Barton created dances with imaginative, sweeping themes: Stocks and Bondage; Art and Artists, where people came as their favorite work of art; Last Night on the Titanic, where members dressed in classy twenties garb; the Brady Bunch Hawaiian Luau, where classy was *not* the point. All the other eating clubs had formal date dances. But since Terrace was alternative-friendly, which included being gay- and lesbian-friendly, the date dances were transformed into wild theme parties.

Terrace was a refuge from the typical Princeton environment. The atmosphere was set by people who didn't want to live by mainstream standards; who had created an identity for themselves based on their creativity, their dissatisfaction with the typical, and their sense of individuality. Here, people could let go of their self-imposed restrictions and just *be*. I liked it. But I couldn't let go of my self-imposed restrictions—not yet.

"Here, dear, chop this. Just chop it coarse, it doesn't need to be too fine." Barton's tall frame was bending over me. His handlebar mustache danced as he told me what to do. Another kitchen worker and I were chopping, Barton and the sous-chef, Chris, were creating, and two other staff members were cleaning. In defiance of its appearance, an old, food-encrusted radio played loud music, setting the rhythm for my work.

"Come here, dear—what's your name? . . . Marianne, look at this menu. I created the whole thing." Barton was showing me the multiple-course meal he had designed for the winter theme party. I had never seen anyone talk about food the way Barton did. His brown eyes locked on to that menu. I could see him tasting the food as he looked at the printed words "Mushrooms stuffed with chopped vegetables in a white wine sauté, Polynesian meatballs, spinach-stuffed lamb roast. . . ." Food was Barton's passion. It was his art. His gift for mixing tastes, textures, colors, and smells gave Barton an outlet, and let him give others pleasure. "The menu looks great, Barton." My voice was weak. I didn't know how to react to Barton's enthusiasm about food because I didn't yet understand food's potential to be a medium of creative expression and a source of individual and social enjoyment.

The night of the party, each room was decorated in the theme of a different artistic movement: impressionism, Renaissance, pop art. Barton put sheets of dot candy at each of about two hundred seats and dyed the rolls pink and green to evoke the artistic style exemplified by Seurat and Signac. I was busy in the kitchen as guests started arriving. Laughter and words melded into a soup of sounds that spilled into the kitchen, which was becoming frenzied and excited. "Here, serve these hors d'oeuvres." I was handed a tray. Going up the stairs, I passed a guy dressed as a Magritte painting with an apple hanging in front of his nose; the left side of his face had a beard and mustache, the right side was clean-shaven. I went into the library and passed a man dressed in drag as Annie Leibovitz, taking pictures of a woman dressed as Marilyn Monroe with a brightly colored face à la Andy Warhol. As I put the tray of cheeses and grapes on the hors d'oeuvres table, I tried not to stare at the human statue: a guy who had put baby powder over his body and stood motionless on the table, naked except for the sheath of whiteness.

At this Terrace party, I was in a role I could handle: working in the kitchen, becoming friends with the kitchen staff, serving food, watching people let go. Watching people dancing and laughing and eating and enjoying. Watching but not quite doing. That was experiencing without risking.

GIVEN MY STRONGER sense of self, I decided to spend the first semester of my senior year in London, interning with a member of Parliament (M.P.) and researching my senior thesis—an independent paper, eighty to one hundred pages in length, that was the culmination of an undergraduate's career at Princeton. I had decided to write my thesis on prostitution. I started with the idea that prostitution was inherently exploitation of women, but after reading some articles and interviewing prostitutes, I changed my position. I began to advocate the legalization of prostitution, with regulations designed to protect the working women from abuse and coercion. Subconsciously, the desire to write about prostitution emerged from my desire to encounter sex at a safe distance. Through my thesis, I could explore sex from an academic, intellectual standpoint, since I was afraid to act on my desire and explore it physically and emotionally.

I binged a lot while I was in London. During my four months there, I missed parties that my colleagues at the M.P.'s office invited me to. I missed them because I needed to binge, or because I felt too fat. But I explored on my own all over London: the Camden Town open-air market; the "red-light" areas like King's Court and Streatham, where I talked with working girls; the "fringe" theaters, which are the British equivalent of off Broadway; the parks. I sometimes wish I had done more with my British friends, but I did all I could have done at the time. In the process, I matured and became better able to connect on a deeper level with those around me and with my environment.

As the months passed, I began to view each of my colleagues as beautiful. Allison, with her stately presence and her statuesque, strong figure; Sophie, a slight nymph with short orange hair and intelligent green eyes; Sarah, with her curly blond hair, wide smile, and angelic blue eyes that engage people directly; Tom, whose view of politics was sure and caring, and whose view of people was the same. As I write this, I feel a need to add a caveat: photographs and media images can strip the meaning from the word "beauty." When I write that my colleagues were beautiful, I write not of typical two-dimensional beauty but of a powerful radiance. They were beautiful not because they fit a standardized image of beauty, but because their spirits and minds and bodies were connected into whole, complete, soulful people.

Before I left Britain, the man I worked for—David Blunkett, a powerful Labour M.P. who was shadow health secretary at the time—took me to lunch in the parliamentary building. I ordered a garden salad, despite David's protest that I should eat more than an appetizer. "I'm just trying to keep my weight down," I said. I didn't tell him I was afraid of eating anything other than salad because I didn't allow myself to eat a hot meal in the middle of the day. Never mind that I would binge later that night.

"Marianne, I'm sure you don't need to lose weight." I laughed nervously, wondering how David could know if I had to lose weight: David is blind. He sensed my nervousness and added, "I can tell you don't need to lose weight by the way you walk and grip my hand, other such things." I sat smiling with David. He creates an image in his mind of what he "sees," just as we all create an image in our minds of what we see. He saw me through the way I walked and gripped his hand; maybe he sees a sunny London day by the warmth on his skin and the smell of the breeze. At that point in my life, I saw myself through the numbers on a scale and the folds on my stomach.

I GOT BACK to Princeton in January; with the pressure to finish my thesis and find a job within the next five months, I needed my bulimia every day. When I binged, I would prowl around the grocery store, tense energy building as I tried to decide on just the right combination of food. *I want the chocolate-covered pretzels with four muffins and a loaf of bread. Wait, no, maybe I want the box of granola and the bagels with cream cheese. But I need something less sweet to cut the granola. . . . But maybe I feel like chocolate. So what should I get that's chocolatey? . . .* I would run through the possibilities as I stood in the cookie aisle, and again as I walked past the ice cream section, and again as my eye focused on peanuts and I started imagining myself eating them, one by one, my hand reaching into the jar and into my mouth over and over. With the possibilities crowding my mind, I would fill the grocery cart with lettuce, tuna fish, apples, whole wheat spaghetti. The low-fat foods had to outnumber the fattening ones in my cart. I had to conceal the fact that I was planning a binge.

I would walk up the aisles conversing silently with myself as my mind jumped from paranoia to anger: *She's looking at my cart. She sees that I'm buying Pepperidge Farm SoftBaked cookies and frozen yogurt. She knows. Damnit, she knows! Well, fuck you, in your little size 6 jeans. Buy your healthy fucking foods, your little lettuce and your little light bread. I'm gonna buy my cookies and I'm gonna eat all of them. ALL OF THEM!*

I would tense up as I waited in the checkout line, in part because I felt guilty and disgusting, in part because I felt the anticipation—the knowledge that I was close to my fix. The food was right there. It was all right there. I would stand at the checkout line, looking around for someone who might know me, thinking, *Come on, come on. This checkout line is so slow. Hurry up, damnit. I need to get out of public with this food. I need to eat this food.* My nerves would shoot off panic, like electricity shooting from an exposed wire.

Sometimes I would go to a couple of stores—bagel shops, bakeries, a grocery store, a frozen yogurt shop. When I got to the cashier, I would smile hard and lie. I would casually mention, "I'll have the bran muffin, but I know Linda likes chocolate, so I'll get her the chocolate muffin, and the other three don't care, so I'll get them . . ." With my forehead creased in concern, I would ask, "Will this cake stay fresh for several days?" knowing that the cake would be gone in an hour. When I ordered pizza over the phone, I would yell into an empty room, *"What? . . . you want spinach? Okay. . . ."* Then I'd calmly say, "We'll have it with spinach topping."

I had many near accidents on the walk or drive home from the stores. Since my mind was focused on the approaching binge, I often failed to notice the cars coming toward me or the pedestrians starting to cross the street. By the time I got safely back to my room during the most intense binges, I was filled with a desperate energy. I would tear into the packaging. My hands would shake. The food was no longer food, it was my drug. It was my lover. I had to devour it.

As I ate, my hands would stop shaking. I would calm down with the first taste of my fix. *Oh, this is so good. This is really fucking good.* I would shovel food into my mouth—one cookie, two cookies, another cookie before I finished chewing the second. I couldn't taste anything now, but tasting wasn't the point. The point was to eat, to chew, to have the sensation of putting food into my mouth. To shut off emotions, to tune out the rules.

I would eventually start to eat more slowly because my stomach didn't want any more. My mouth would grow dry. But I would put food into my mouth, chewing, swallowing, thirsting for water. *Keep eating. . . . But I can't. I'm stuffed, it doesn't taste good, my stomach hurts. I can't eat. . . . Eat it, Marianne.* The food would overflow my stomach and rest high in my chest. But I would force myself to keep eating. *Finish it, Marianne. After today, you won't ever pig out again. You won't let yourself eat a whole box of cereal again, so enjoy it now. Finish it. . . . But I'm sick. My stomach hurts. I can't eat any more. . . . Eat it.* I would chew slowly because I didn't think I could make myself swallow. I didn't think I could eat anymore. That's when I would make myself throw up.

I would work my way to the bathroom, my body bent slightly at the waist because the food pulled my upper body down. When I got to the bathroom, I would mechanically wash my right index finger, crouch over the toilet, and stick my finger deep into my throat. Sometimes it was easy. Undigested, barely chewed food would fall from me into the toilet. As the wave of food moved through my body, I would surge, body arching from the force of the angry purge. My belly would contract hard, my back would curve like a frightened cat's, my knees would become anchored to the cold tile floor. After each wave, I would dry my hand and dive back into my throat for another wave. A few minutes later, I wouldn't be able to do it again. My body would hurt. Droplets of vomit and toilet water would cling to my face and chest. For a few minutes, unsettled energy would eat at my ears like insects. I would wash off the vomit, brush my teeth, and climb out of the bathroom. My heart would be beating fast. The smell of vomit—that delicate, sweet, repulsive smell—would linger on my index finger for hours.

I wouldn't be able to process my behavior right away. I would usually sleep, my eyes stinging and puffy. I slept from the physical exhaustion of having forced my body to accept and reject mounds of food, and from the emotional exhaustion of having felt that I would never be free of my bulimia and my sadness. But I wouldn't feel sad at that moment. I would feel detached, distant from my emotions and my body. I was at rest.

Later, after I woke up and saw my swollen belly in the mirror, smelled the vomit in the bathroom, stepped over the dirty dishes—then I would cry or rage in self-disgust. *How could I be so gross? Just stop. Why can't I just stop? I should just stop, damnit. What is wrong with you, Marianne? What's WRONG with you!* And the energy would build, and the feelings would intensify, and I would soon eat again.

THROUGHOUT MY LAST semester at Princeton, I rocked from that kind of binge eating to anorexic eating, back and forth, weight building and weight shrinking. Usually the anorexic eating lasted a couple of days at most. But on a couple of occasions, I dieted for several weeks. I watched with a sense of power as my belly stopped swelling. The jeans that had hung lifeless in the closet slid onto my body, taking the form of my rounded hips and strong legs. When I felt this way, I went to Terrace with friends at night, created opportunities for myself to have a good time. As expected, I had more fun when I went out with friends than when I stayed home by myself eating. I attributed the increase in happiness and self-confidence to the weight loss. I was wrong. The difference was in self-perception: it wasn't in the way I looked, but in the way I *felt* about the way I looked.

When I wasn't bingeing, I liked the way I looked with curves. Feminine, sultry, strong, confident. I experienced the power of a woman's body—the power to attract, feel desire, have fun, express empathy, soothe. I could dance and exercise with this body. I could embrace a friend and smile at a stranger with this body. I could wear tight shirts that hugged my breasts, low-cut blouses that accentuated my curves.

But that confidence never lasted long, because it was based on beliefs that weren't accurate: namely, that I could use willpower to overcome a coping mechanism I had relied on for years, and that everything would fall into place once I lost some weight. Even when I was in the "high" of dieting, I somehow knew that I hadn't released myself from my obsession with food and body. I somehow knew that I would go back to bingeing because I hadn't dealt with the reasons behind my eating disorder. The knowledge that the sexy and confident feelings wouldn't last gave those feelings an urgency. I had to take advantage of them *now*. I had to do everything *now*. I had to explore *now*, because soon—I didn't know when, but definitely soon—this feeling would be gone and I would be fat and sad again.

With that mind-set, I started sleeping around. I didn't let myself get involved much beyond one-night physical relationships because I was afraid to let someone see the whole of my personality—afraid to feel the emotional openness and vulnerability that come with an intimate relationship. I was also afraid of the physical aspects of a relationship. I couldn't deal with the concept of a man touching my body or seeing me naked for more than one night. I thought that if I gained weight, I would disappoint him, become the object of his disgust, make myself vulnerable to his mockery and rejection. How could a man see my belly after a binge? How could I feel sexy if I was thinking about sucking in my stomach and getting rid of the taste of vomit in my mouth?

Yet despite my fears about entering a deep relationship, I was a woman who, when I wasn't bingeing, felt the beauty of her body and a natural sexual desire. I was also an insecure woman who thought that sex could prove my body was okay. So during my senior year, after two years of kissing and mildly fooling around occasionally, "relationships" became a series of one-night stands.

At first, that kind of physical intimacy felt fantastic. After years of telling myself I was disgusting and unattractive, I was thrilled by the charge of seduction, the newness of sex, my uncharacteristic boldness with men. But after four or five of these little flings, I started to understand that the ability to attract men for one-nighters was an empty power. The sex had no substance. It became dull. The physical act wasn't joined with a deeply meaningful emotion—caring, shared openness, love, the exhilaration of mutual trust. Instead it was joined with a cognitive device: the need to prove to myself that I could be seductive and attractive, the need to get some confirmation of my worth as a woman. I couldn't give myself over to the state of release, the state of pure feeling, because I didn't trust the men I was with, I didn't love them, and I didn't care for them. I just wanted to have sex with them when I could—when I felt attractive—before the carriage turned back into a pumpkin, the white horses into mice, and the sexy Marianne into the bulimic Marianne.

Eventually, the binges on sex would lead back to binges on food because I hadn't dealt with the reasons for my self-doubt and self-hate, and because losing weight and attracting men

weren't miracle cures for my unhappiness. Physically, I could-
n't withstand the starvation diet, either. My body needed more
food than I was giving it. The break back to bingeing always
started with just a bit of food. *Fuck, Marianne, why did you eat
that piece of bread?!* . . . *Well, that's fine, I just ate bread, I won't
eat anymore.* . . . *Well, maybe a cup of dry cereal.* . . . Another
cup. A third. *I'm going to the store. Damnit!* I had a sense of res-
ignation, of "here we go again," back to the bingeing Marianne.

After one typical cycle in which desperate exploration ended
in desperate eating, I started pacing the floor strewn with wrappers, empty cartons, dirty plates. That morning I had worn a
short black skirt and a scooped-neck top. I had felt good walking through campus; I'd walked with a sense of confidence, a
sense that I was a woman, a strong woman, an interesting
woman. Now, hours later, I was disgusting again. I was ugly and
incompetent and pathetic again. BOOM, BOOM, BOOM.
My right fist slammed against the wall. Over and over. BOOM,
BOOM, BOOM. I needed to hurt myself. I needed to hurt this
body that had betrayed me. *You're fat, Marianne. YOU'RE
FAT. You looked good this morning and now you're FAT. You
deserve it, Marianne. You deserve to sit home with your food and
your fatness!* BOOM, BOOM, BOOM. *Marianne, why did you
ruin it? Why?*

# S I X

■

# Falling Exhausted

# into Therapy

I WAS tired. I had spent six years telling myself to stop bingeing, and berating myself when I failed. Up and down, all or none. I had spent six years telling myself the bulimia would get better once I got to college, once freshman year was over, once I was an upperclassman, once I graduated. And it never got better. In January of senior year, I came to accept what I had known for a long time. The eating disorder wouldn't go away on its own, it wouldn't go away through willpower, it wouldn't go away with a change of scenery. I needed professional help. That January, I fell exhausted into therapy because I had no strength to do anything else.

The tight skin of the apple broke as I devoured my breakfast and sucked its light, sweet juices. The new diet was sparked by my appointment with Theresa, a psychologist at Princeton's health clinic. Today was the first day of therapy, and despite my initial misgivings, I was excited. I was ready to conquer my eating disorder. This was it. No more bulimia. Theresa could make me thin; she would give me a concrete plan to follow so I'd never binge again. After all, I thought, since the whole point of therapy was to eliminate the bulimia, it would be ludicrous for me to binge and go to a therapist at the same time.

As I walked toward the clinic in McCosh Hall, my excitement evaporated. *Does anyone see me? Will they see me walk in? Will anyone know I'm going to therapy?* I moved closer to the building, watching, scanning the walkways for people I knew, for people who might catch me entering the mental health clinic.

"Hi. Do you have an appointment?" The receptionist smiled. I hated her for smiling. Did she think I would crack up if she treated me normally? "Yes. Ten o'clock with Theresa." The receptionist led me down the hall. She was wearing a long skirt that flowed off her hips, floral pattern fluttering. *She's thin. See, I need to be thin like that. Just like her.* "Theresa should be with you soon," she said as she shut the door, creating an echo of sound that moved through the room. I sat still on a small couch, nerves alert, until Theresa's figure entered.

*Great. Just great. This woman is fat. I'm supposed have some overweight woman tell me how to put food in perspective! She's supposed to tell me how to lose weight! What am I doing here? She should get control of herself before she tells me how to get control. What am I doing here?* My reaction to Theresa was hateful and nasty. I needed those hard emotions; they were a defense against my sense that I was diseased and pathetic for going to therapy. As my relationship with Theresa developed that day and later that year, I would come to see her as a powerful and beautiful African-American woman with a strong sense of herself and a concern for other people.

I hadn't realized that yet. Now I just felt anger and fear. I sat on the couch across from Theresa's chair. A small table holding a box of tissues stood between us. I looked at those tissues.

*What are those here for? I'm not going to cry. Do you expect us all to cry? We're not all weak.* I felt suspicious. I was a guinea pig in their little game of therapy. I didn't want to be there.

Theresa asked about the basics—my age, family structure, eating patterns. We hadn't gotten much further when I reached for one of those tissues to twist in my hand and dry my eyes. For eight years, I had never spoken with anyone about my eating disorder. It was such a release to talk about it without fear of judgment, to say with words and emotions: "I've been hurting, I don't want to be hurting so much anymore." To say: "*Help me.*"

But the kind of help I wanted from Theresa was different from what good therapists, including Theresa, were offering. I wanted therapy to be my new Diet Center. It would give me answers as to why I was bingeing, just as the Diet Center had given me answers as to what foods I should eat. Therapy would provide a specific plan designed to stop the behavior, just as the Diet Center had provided a specific plan designed to help me lose weight. I would be accountable to my therapist: she would know if I had binged, she would see if I followed the suggestions she gave me, if I improved. I would be accountable to her, just as I had been accountable to that perky woman at the Diet Center who asked me to step on the scale each Saturday morning. That would stop me from bingeing: the answers, the plan, the need for my counselor's approval. It was simple.

Simple and wrong. When I started therapy, I thought of my eating disorder in terms of food, not in terms of emotions. I didn't realize that therapy would only be effective if I dealt with the purpose bingeing served for me; sought an alternative and healthier way of serving that purpose; and modified the thinking/feeling/acting patterns that created my need for a release in food. The point of therapy is to put an end to the *symptoms* of an eating disorder—the starvation, bingeing, and/or purging— but only by dealing with the fundamental *causes* of those symptoms.

At my second session, Theresa asked evenly, "Okay, Marianne, you're saying you won't eat cookies and muffins until you're down to the weight you want to be at. But what would happen if you let yourself have a cookie when you want to have a cookie?" What was she saying! My fingers curled around the cushioned arm of the chair. My back pushed deep into the back of my seat as my body tensed and my face froze in a half smile. I was threatened by the question *"What would happen if you let yourself have a cookie when you want to have a cookie?"* To me, that wasn't a valid question. The thought of eating a fattening food in moderation was incompatible with the structure I had developed to make sense of myself and my environment: I was supposed to have control over my food. No fattening foods. I must have control.

"I don't know what would happen. But I don't think I really need cookies right now. Maybe in a few weeks or something." *Marianne, don't listen to her. I am not going to eat cookies anytime I want to.* "I just, I mean, I don't want to eat sweets right now. Like, not till I lose some weight first, you know? Then I'll try that." Even though my voice sounded somewhat open to Theresa's suggestion, my tightened muscles told her: *I can't do it, Theresa. Don't ask me to do it, Theresa, please!*

At the time of this session, I couldn't appreciate the freedom and power Theresa was offering me. She was telling me that nothing was stopping me from eating. No one was passing judgment. No one was saying I would be a better person if I ate no fat. If I want a bagel with loads of cream cheese, I should buy it. If I want a chocolate fudge brownie, I should eat one. Theresa was letting me know that I had the power to choose. Unlike those diets that tell you you're "good" if you stick to a regimented food plan and "bad" if you don't, Theresa was giving *me* the authority to listen to what my body wanted and needed. She was also telling me that if I took the "charge" out of eating—if I removed the elements of judgment and self-denigration that accompanied eating—I could weaken the grip bulimia had on me. It took me several years to grasp and implement that idea.

Session three. "Now, Marianne, what would happen if you went to Terrace on a night when you binged?" Again, Theresa's question challenged my philosophy: I let myself experience only when I had lost weight.

"What would happen if I went to Terrace on a night I binged? I'd be uncomfortable. I wouldn't be able to move, I'd feel, like, weighted down and sick."

"Is that based on experience? Have you done that?"

"Yeah, well, no, not actually on the day I binged."

"Um-hmm."

"I went out a few weeks ago, when Terrace had Greek Night and they had a band come in and we did Greek dancing, which was really fun. But I hadn't binged for at least, like, two days before that."

"So you had fun?"

"Yeah, but I hadn't binged that day."

"No, but you also didn't get down to your 'goal weight.' "

"Uh-huh." I was beginning to resent her again. Where did she get off trying to create my social calendar? *I don't need a social planner, thank you.*

Theresa had no interest in becoming my social planner. But she knew that I was trying to leave behind my eating disorder before letting myself feel pleasure; she also knew that I had to feel pleasure—feel emotions that were more satisfying than the numbness of bulimia—before I could leave behind my eating disorder.

The session continued. "Have you ever tried to sit with feelings, Marianne?"

*Sit with feelings? I feel too much! That's the point! I need to stop feeling, and you want me to sit with feelings?!* "I don't, I don't know what you mean."

"Sometimes, if you don't try to stop a feeling, it will pass on its own, and you'll realize that you can move on. No feeling stays with you always."

"Fine. I'll try that." My words were sharp. I had thought that I was somehow different, that I was somehow a "superfeeler" — exceptionally passionate and emotionally in touch. Now Theresa was saying I suppressed my emotions, that I felt them strongly on a surface level but did not let them sink into me where I could hold them and process them.

"Do you like to take baths? Maybe you could take a bath and soothe yourself. You could take a bath and sit with your emotions without trying to get rid of them. Or go for a walk. You've said several times you like to go for walks."

"Um, yeah, uh-huh." I was making her work. I resisted her suggestions because they threatened me: "sit with feelings" and "walk to soothe yourself" were suggestions I knew I could not yet follow. Yet I was a woman who had always followed the rules, who didn't want to disappoint her therapist, and who had convinced herself that specific suggestions from a professional would eliminate the eating disorder. Instead of discussing my discomfort with Theresa, my muscles and emotions got hard.

"Okay, Marianne, well that's one idea that will keep coming up, that idea of sitting with feelings and being able to *feel* them rather than push them down and numb yourself out."

"Okay." I was glad Theresa didn't press the point and went on to another line of discussion. But I knew we had been talking about something important, something I couldn't avoid.

At the end of a few individual sessions, Theresa suggested I join Princeton's eating disorders therapy group. My muscles drooped tired and my mind moved slow as if to say, "Fine, if you say group therapy will help, I'll try group therapy." Two weeks later I walked into the therapy room and smelled fear and weakness. I hated those eight people sitting in a circle. I hated them because they were a mirror of me: in their fear and weakness, I saw my own. "Okay, let's introduce ourselves," began Betty, who was the counselor and facilitator of the group, along with Theresa.

I had already introduced myself with my body—lips pursed, arms folded, legs crossed. The knotted tightness of my body told the group I was not going to share, I was not going to be touchy-feely, I had no compassion for myself or them. "Don't touch me," my body said. "You can see the prickles on my skin, you can see that I will hurt you if you touch me. So leave me alone."

If the group members didn't hear the message in my body language, they heard it in my words. "I'm Marianne, and I'm a senior in the politics department, and I'll be graduating in a few months, thank God. And I've been anorexic for two years and bulimic for six. And I was seeing Theresa for a while and she suggested I come to group. And so I'm here. And I'm cynical that this can do anything. I don't think that sitting and talking with a group of strangers can stop me from shoving food in my face and sticking my finger down my throat. . . . And I'm angry because I don't want to be here. This whole thing makes me feel really weak. And I'm not a weak person . . . or, I mean, I don't see myself as a weak person. And now I feel really weak, and I hate people who are weak. It's like, 'Get a fucking grip on yourself, Marianne. Stop shoving food in your mouth and get a fucking grip.' . . . So that's my shtick."

Everyone else introduced themselves a lot less harshly. There was an intelligent woman who had had a short bout with bulimia, but who was now fairly stable; a freshman actor with a sweet demeanor; a senior who taught aerobics and had a job lined up in the catering business; a tomboy freshman in the "in" crowd; a black woman who was a member of one of Princeton's elite a cappella singing groups; and one male, a runner who was soft-spoken and sincere.

Over the next ninety minutes, we talked, learned a bit about one another, exchanged stories about moments of embarrass-

ment and sadness and hurt. As we talked, my defense mechanism—the wall of anger that protected me from fear and self-
hate—broke under the force of compassion and sadness. At first
it was easier to be callous than to let myself feel my unhappiness. But the unhappiness was in me at my core, and as the participants shared their stories, thoughts, and feelings, I began to
feel those core emotions. They filled my body, making me want
to hug my knees to my chest and cry.

Toward the end of the session, Theresa asked, "Marianne,
how do you feel about the group after this first session?"

Sigh. "I'm not as cynical. And I'm not as angry. And . . . um,
I'm still skeptical that all this can make a difference, but . . ." I
stopped speaking as I looked down at my feet. I didn't want to
share the other words that were coming to mind: "How did I
end up here? Will I ever be done with this? I don't want to analyze and probe anymore, I just want to be *done* with this. I want
to be normal. I want it to go away. . . . Can you make it go away?
Can you do that? Will it ever go away?"

The session ended. We had been talking for over an hour
about secret, intimate things; but after we left the room, none
of us shared a word of comfort or a pleasantry or the standard
"see you next week." We walked in silence out of McCosh Hall
and scattered toward our separate existences.

I was walking home at the end of the second group session,
my mind wandering as I moved. *Those people sitting around the
circle aren't my friends. But I tell them feelings I've never told
anyone else. What am I doing there? Do I trust them? Do they
care about me? Do I care about them?* Passing the library, where
I had read and searched and binged and thrown up, I questioned the concept of group therapy even more. *Can I relate to
those people? We all have an eating disorder. So we relate. . . .
But our world isn't just our eating disorder, is it? I don't want to
be pigeonholed because of my behavior. I don't want to be
labeled bulimic. I don't want my eating disorder to be who I am!*

As I reached the main street, my emotions were gathering in my throat, wanting to tumble out of me, wanting to exhaust themselves. But instead of crying, I turned right on the main street, entered a store, and ordered a bagel. "You know what, just throw on a bunch of that cinnamon cream cheese. . . . And my roommates like your muffins. . . . Do you have any of those this afternoon?"

Having had two months of individual and group therapy, I still needed to swallow my emotions, to push them down from my throat to my stomach since I couldn't release them through words or tears. During therapy, I had come to realize that my emotions wouldn't exhaust themselves in the binge/purge—not the way they would if I felt them in my throat, my body, my mouth as I cried. During therapy, I had come to realize that part of my emotions would be ripped from me as I ripped the food from my stomach, and part would hide inside me, stunned into numbness from the battering of food and ready to stir once the numbness wore off. Despite therapy and the knowledge I gained from it, I binged. Letting go is a long process.

I learned most from the group during the fourth session. "Do you know how many times you said 'should' in the last half hour?" One group member was looking at me.

"What?" I was startled. I felt trapped, like I'd done something wrong.

"You say 'should' a lot, like you have these expectations of the way everything should be."

My cheeks tingled as embarrassment grabbed hold of my face and body.

"That's an interesting point." Theresa was weighing in now.

*Okay, fine, just keep it up, guys, just keep piling it on.* I felt like they were ganging up on me, harping on my faults, adding to the list of things I did wrong. But my body and mind were hyperaware, holding tight to their words and insights.

"It's like you put this pressure on yourself to achieve these, like, totally unrealistic goals."

"Maybe your expectations are so high that you're always setting yourself up for disappointment or failure or something."

After that session, I began noticing the s word—noticing how that word, that concept, saturated my speech. I *should* be over this bulimia. I *should* have a job. I *should* get an A on my thesis. I *should* control my food. I *should* have a boyfriend. I *should* be prettier. I *should* make Phi Beta Kappa. If I wasn't everything I *should* be, I was an absolute failure. All or none.

It was helpful to hear the insights of group members, and to share insights, too, when I had the opportunity. By listening to one another—by helping another person work through her/his problems—we were acquiring skills that would be useful in dealing with our own problems. By helping another person, we were teaching ourselves new ways to think, feel, and act. It was powerful to be able to help another person who was hurting in a way I understood. And it was powerful to realize I had the ability to help myself, just as I had the ability to help her.

But group therapy was hard, and I wasn't used to its rawness. I felt uncomfortable at times, witnessing a group member stand naked without her defenses, her emotions and actions exposed. I felt each person's humanness. They were good people who had faced daunting situations: physical or emotional abuse; responsibilities too great for a child; ultrahigh expectations; unhealthy family dynamics with siblings, mother, father, stepparent, etc. They were people who dealt with those situations with strength. But such exertions created a vacuum in their spirit—a vacuum in their sense of self. And like me, they shrank the vacuum by shrinking their body, or filled the vacuum by filling their body with food. Like me, they were trying to fill a vacuum of the *spirit* by changing the shape of their *body*.

They were not weak. They were strong, surviving in the best

way they knew how. As I started to feel compassion for them, I started to feel compassion for myself: I am not a disgusting, awful person because I do this. I am a person with a problem, just as they are people with problems, just as we are all people with problems. This newfound compassion for myself gave me space to travel forward on my path, even if I still binged. By the end of the last session, I felt comfortable saying that bulimia was my coping mechanism. For so many years I had never said the word "bulimia," never let those sounds pass through my lips: "bu-lim-i-a." Each week in group therapy, I formed that word, and I became comfortable with the notion that I wasn't a freak because I was bulimic.

Therapy helped me find the words and compassion that enabled me to share my secret with friends and family. I could tell them about my struggles, I could ask them for help and support and love. By letting go of the secret and freeing myself from the burden of guilt, I was able to focus my energy on changing, not on perpetuating the lie.

I WAS BREAKING down. My thesis wasn't coming together. I had two weeks left and the thing was a monster: too long, too unfocused, too loose, flabby, oversized. I didn't have a job, but classmates around me were being hired at consulting firms, law firms, investment banking companies; they were getting into law school, med school, Ph.D. programs. I had résumés at fifteen different TV news departments and documentary production companies. Nothing. No response. Except one letter saying I hadn't made the final round of interviews.

Waves of food pounded into my stomach until my stomach rejected them. I watched the cursor of my computer wink at me, mocking me as I attempted to revise my thesis. I biked hard, pushing, sweating, moving nowhere on the exercise bike at the gym. I listened to excited descriptions of new graduate programs to be started in the fall. I felt my mouth twitch as classmates with overconfident faces told of their new jobs, for which they had been courted aggressively.

One night I called George. "George, I'm, like, I don't know what I'm doing. I can't even, I mean my thesis is thirty pages too long, and it's just huge, and I don't know, I don't know if I can cut it down or make it work or . . ." I was crying even before he had picked up the phone. "And I don't even have a job. How could I work so hard and not have a job? All these little shits who never did any of the assigned reading, who showed up in class and had nothing to say—they all have jobs. I don't have a job. And I worked so hard. I worked so hard here, I don't understand. . . . I didn't even go out on the weekends. I stayed home and worked. . . . Why did I do that? Why did I waste so much time working? . . ." My voice was barely audible through the tears.

"I know, I know." George was hurting. I could hear in his voice that he wanted to help me.

"And I binge all the time! I'm so fat now! I binge and eat and stuff my face, and then I go to the bathroom and make myself throw up. . . . I feel so sad, I'm so sad, George."

"Oh, Mare. . . ."

"I can't help it, I try so hard to help it, I can't. . . . I try so hard. . . ."

"Sometimes . . . I know this might sound weird to you, but sometimes if you pray at night, just to calm yourself down and think about things a little . . . sometimes that helps."

"No, no . . ." I was wailing. "No, no, it's too big, it's too much. . . . Praying won't help, no, no, no." I was making him uncomfortable. With each wail, I was withdrawing from the "normal" state of consciousness and approaching a state of hysteria, where all my defenses were exhausted, where I was letting my confusion spill out untamed. With each of my steps into hysteria, George was becoming more and more grounded in the normal state of consciousness, and more and more desperate to bring me back.

"Mare, I mean, have you tried . . . have you tried to, like, just stop eating . . . ?" He knew it was the wrong thing to say. But he needed to help me. And he needed to help himself—to stop the discomfort I was causing him.

*Just stop eating.* That phrase brought me back to my normal state of consciousness. Just stop eating. My defenses shot back, I bottled my emotions and became presentable. "Maybe I'll try those things, but right now I really have to get working again on this thesis. Thanks, George, for letting me talk to you and everything, and just, you know . . ."

"You sure you're okay? . . . I don't want to let you off the phone until you're okay."

"Yeah, I'm fine. I'm just stressed out because of my dumb thesis. But I'll be fine, I got it out of my system."

"Are you sure you're okay? I mean, I don't want to let you go until—"

"I'm fine." My voice was firm.

"Okay. But call me *anytime* you need to. You know, just to talk or whatever."

"Okay. Bye, George. Thanks."

Just stop eating. He had tried to help the best way he knew how. He had tried to give me advice about how to stop. It wasn't the advice I needed. I felt alone. I felt he had belittled my emotions, invalidated the intensity I had felt for eight years. That night, I didn't realize what a difficult situation I had put my brother in, I didn't realize that he would need time to learn about bulimia and learn how to give support. That night, I just felt that the person I admired most, the person who had helped me more than anyone, didn't understand and couldn't help me anymore. My support was gone and I was alone. He told me to stop eating. As if it were the simplest thing in the world.

I dragged myself to the stereo, changed CDs, and sat on the floor. I huddled into a ball and rocked back and forth. Nirvana's *In Utero* played loud in the background, camouflaging the sounds of my screams. After a while, when I couldn't cry any-more, I got my car keys and drove to the supermarket to buy food for a binge. Just stop eating, he'd said.

I told my parents in a similar way—over the phone in a moment after a binge when I was feeling the fear of leaving Princeton and moving to Manhattan. They too tried to give pat responses and easy solutions. But that was okay; at that point, I was just glad we had killed the secret.

# PART
# FOUR

■

# I'm Satisfied

S   E   V   E   N

■

# Exploration

FTER months of searching for work, I fell into a job
as a research associate at a Manhattan-based drug policy
research institute run by a former Princeton professor. My colleagues argued that our current drug policy is more about pun-
ishment and control than about caring and autonomy. Through
my conversations and reading, I began to understand and agree
with their perspective. I also began to see my colleagues as independent thinkers who had created their own paradigm for the
way they wanted to live. I began to see myself as that kind of person, too. I began to understand who I wanted to be.

Because of my work, I spent time at several needle exchanges
and their affiliated harm reduction centers in New York City.
Needle exchanges help to reduce the spread of HIV, hepatitis,
and other infections by providing clean needles to people with
heroin or cocaine addictions when they bring their dirty needles
in for safe disposal. The exchanges embrace the idea that even

if clients are poor, unclean, or addicted to drugs, they are people deserving of human contact and caring. In addition to providing clean needles and referrals to detoxification and drug
treatment programs, some exchanges provide medical treatment, social services, support groups, acupuncture, and other
therapies.

While I was at the exchanges, I felt like I knew a bit about
what the clients were feeling. I didn't know the fear of the law,
the poverty, or the intensity of physical and psychological with-
drawal symptoms from heroin or cocaine. These factors put the
needle-exchange clients at a tremendous disadvantage relative
to me. But I did know the need to numb out, the need to lose
this reality. I knew the guilt, the embarrassment, the continuous
efforts to convince myself that this was it, the last time, the very
last time, tomorrow I will come clean. By connecting with people at the needle exchanges, I deepened my sense of compassion for people with addictive behaviors, whether the behavior
revolved around heroin or tobacco or food. The parallels
between drug addiction and eating disorders became more evi-
dent each night as I worked on a manuscript about eating disorders. That manuscript eventually evolved into the words you
are reading now.

Despite the positive aspects of my job and the interest of
W. W. Norton in my manuscript, I felt overwhelmed.
Manhattan towered over me, boxed me in. I absorbed its nervous energy and added it to my own. People were all around
me—pushing against me on the subways, banging against me
on the crowded sidewalks, ruining the illusion of a peaceful
countryside in Central Park—but I felt alone. I was sharing
physical space with them, not emotional space. I had left my
tight group of friends for 8 million strangers.

After a few weeks in New York, I began to feel afraid of
myself, afraid of my compulsion to make myself numb when I
was alone. I created distractions: I would go to the movies, see

a play, walk in Central Park, meet friends downtown. But the distractions were temporary, and I would always be left alone with myself. That's when I would banish all thoughts and emotions and binge more than I ever had before.

By the wintertime, I decided that I needed to see a therapist again. As the N/R subway rode farther downtown, the crowd thinned out. The look of my fellow passengers changed: fewer suits and high-heeled shoes, more piercings and heavy black boots. The heel of my foot, trapped in a three-inch-heeled shoe, started bobbing up and down, fast and nervous. I got off the subway at Prince Street and wandered around Houston Street until I found the dirty building where my therapist worked. After a few minutes' wait, the double doors of my therapist's office opened, and a woman walked out crying. As she passed by, a second woman spoke. "Marianne? Hi, good to see you. Come right in."

The room was dark. The most intense light seemed to emanate from the red numbers on a digital clock. The sounds of the street—the honking, screeching, talking—filled the room. *What am I doing here!*

"Marianne, before we begin I'd like you to fill out this questionnaire." It was a standard depression/suicide questionnaire: "Do you think about killing yourself? If so, how often? Have you ever tried to kill yourself? How many hours a day do you sleep?" etc., etc. Then there was a "getting to know you" section: age, name of family members, age of family members, etc. The therapist and that form alienated me. I wanted a safe space, a comfortable space, to open up and dig deeper. Instead I got a multiple-choice test. I wanted her to talk with me, to show me she could help me in ways my friends couldn't, even though my friends didn't need a questionnaire to know I had a brother.

After her perusal of the form, we talked for fifty minutes. "Well, Marianne, this was a good start. I suggest you start a food journal this week, where you write down what you eat. We can go over it next week and learn some patterns from it." I said nothing. The therapist didn't ask me if I was ready to keep a food journal, she didn't ask how I felt about the idea. At this stage, the journal would have passed judgment on me each time I ate. It would have become my tyrant, and I would have made it so. But the therapist didn't seem concerned about that.

She asked one final question before I left: Do I want to keep this day and this hour to come each week for therapy? "You know what, I don't know what my schedule will be like. Let me give you a call." I wrote the check, left the office, got swallowed by the subway, and got spit out uptown. I never saw her again.

Since that day, several people have told me it's a good idea to see a therapist two or three times before deciding whether to stay with her/him. That's a valid suggestion, because people often have apprehensions about going to therapy, and those apprehensions can negatively color a first impression. But sometimes a client can separate the apprehension she brings to therapy from the ones arising from the style of the therapist. In this case, I trusted myself: I didn't like the style of the therapist, and I didn't go back.

A few months later I tried therapy again, getting a referral from my mother's friend who is a therapist. Off I went one more time in search of the "cure." I got a much better feeling from this new therapist, who was less insistent and more relaxed than the other woman. I was gaining an outlet for my feelings and thoughts, and a greater understanding of my behavior.

Donna and I talked about my childhood and adolescence. "It seems like George was hard to live up to." George—I had never thought of George as someone who had influenced my development. But Donna's analysis made total sense: I constantly compared myself to George, I measured myself against the benchmarks of his success. He wasn't to blame for my eating disorder, but he had played an important role in my development. Donna and I also discussed my current binge/purge patterns: what did I do beforehand, how did I feel beforehand, how did I feel afterward? "It seems that you binge sometimes to stop the loneliness. You say you eat after you come home from a movie with friends, in a way to stop the feeling of separation." Okay, yes, that made sense, too. But Donna gave me very little practical advice. I didn't know what to do with the insights I'd gained. I didn't know how to use my new knowledge to help me deal with the bingeing.

In addition, Donna's style was making me increasingly uncomfortable. She would often sit without saying anything, waiting for me to bring up a subject or reveal how I was truly feeling, as if the silence would cause me to say what was *really* on my mind. During one session, when we were sitting in the tiny room looking at each other in silence, I finally blurted, "What do you want me to say?" "Whatever is on your mind, Marianne." *What's on my mind is that I want to get up and leave.*

At the time, I didn't know that Donna's style of directing therapy wasn't the only choice available, and that it was okay for me to want a different kind of therapist. Some people respond to Donna's style, others don't; we each have to shop around until we find the therapist who best meets our needs.

MY COUSIN SOPHIA, who is a musician in several ethnic bands, picked me up at the Toronto airport. I could see her untamed black hair as I approached the baggage area. Even though I hadn't spoken with Sophia or her husband John since their wedding four years earlier, I had always felt a latent connection with them. I felt we would establish that connection when we were ready. Now that I had graduated from college, we were ready.

We went to their friend Rick's house, where people were gathering to celebrate the premiere of a TV show starring their friend Anna. When we arrived, Rick was stirring a pot of rata-touille. We were standing in his kitchen, surrounded by garlic cloves, dirty plates, a mixture of fresh, sharp smells. As I met the circle of people gathering there that night, I realized that Sophia and her friends had created their own community of people who cared about one another, about their society, about finding beauty around them. I found myself feeling at ease with this group of people. As we talked, I was not aware of looks, I was not engaged in constant comparisons with other women. Instead, I was immersed in the moment.

A few weeks later I got a call from Rick. When he said he was coming to New York for the weekend, my body released a slight surge of the sense of wholeness I'd experienced in Toronto. The more time I spent with Rick that weekend, the more I was attract-ed to his intelligence and vulnerability, to his cologne and mouth and aura of sexuality. We went to dinner at a vegetarian restaurant on Manhattan's Lower East Side, where we split a rice pudding sundae for dessert. I scooped up a bit of the sundae, slowly put it in my mouth, let Rick see my tongue lick the last drop of sweetness off the spoon. I wasn't thinking about calories. I wasn't calculating. I was eating and talking and laughing. Later that night Rick kissed me. That was the first time I felt comfort-able kissing a man. Throughout all my one-night stands, I hard-ly kissed a man's lips. I didn't want to: I didn't want to get too close to the *person*; I was focusing only on the *body*. That night, waiting for a taxi outside the Sweet Basil jazz club, I kissed Rick, and my body and self opened to the touch of his lips.

Rick went back to Toronto, we wrote to each other and spoke on the phone, and I tried not to binge. Why would I need to binge? *An incredible guy is interested in me, I have a cool job, I'm living in Manhattan. I'm doing everything I said I wanted to do, I have everything I said I needed to make me happy. Why am I still unhappy? Why do I still find such comfort in food? Comfort from what?*

I didn't realize until later that my whole thought process—
the whole way in which I viewed myself and my relationships
with others and my environment—was the problem. Not the
specific situation I was in, not the specific content of what was
going on in my life. There's no question that a specific situation
can make things better or worse, but I create my own reality: I
create the way I deal with work, with relationships, with myself
and my body. Nothing external can change that—not having a
boyfriend, not getting a good job, not living in an exciting city.
Something internal needed to change: I needed to change my
patterns of thinking and feeling and acting.

I didn't fully realize this idea at the time. In the first month
after Rick came to New York, I fell into a consistent pattern: I
restricted my eating to be sure I looked good for him and felt
good about myself; after feeling deprived and dissatisfied and
hungry, I binged and purged for a couple of days; then I forced
myself to stop bingeing and think about how I wanted to please
Rick, be pleased by him, and have a strong relationship.

I occasionally talked with Rick about my eating disorder. But
I always talked about it when I was in control. I may have said
I was bulimic, but I never let him know me as a person with
bulimia. I never shared with him the state of urgency I felt
before a binge, or the self-disgust I felt after a purge. I may have
been expressing a vulnerability to Rick, but I was never making
myself vulnerable.

The box of granola was on the floor next to the bagel wrapper. My mouth was dry. I felt sad and angry. Mostly sad.

*Ring. . . . I'm not gonna get it.*

*Ring. . . . I'm not gonna get it.*

*Ring.* "Hello?"

"Hi, Marianne. It's Rick." He sounded sexy with his clipped
voice. For a moment I imagined his mouth talking into the
phone. But my mind quickly came back to my stomach. We
talked for a while. We had phone sex. I heard him coming. I

made noises, like I was into it, but my focus was on the monologue in my mind: *Marianne, you can't binge anymore. You're
dating now. When he comes to New York in two weeks, you'll
turn him off. He'll get disgusted. He'll think you're ugly and fat.
. . . You're an ugly and fat kid, Marianne! Stop bingeing,
Marianne! STOP BINGEING!* When we got off the phone, I
went to the bathroom to undo the damage I had done with the
granola and bagel.

When Rick came to visit in December, my body was tense,
and he felt it. I was constantly concerned about my weight,
worried I would disappoint Rick, afraid I would have to put an
immediate end to my bulimia in order to continue dating.
Unconsciously, I told myself I had to choose between bulimia
and Rick. I chose bulimia.

That "all or none" choice was false. I could have talked with
Rick about my bulimia, tried to work on it while we were
together. But I didn't give myself that middle-ground choice. As
a result, I made it impossible to stay with Rick because it was
impossible to give up, immediately, a coping mechanism I had
relied on for eight years. So I pushed Rick away before we could
get close. I didn't want anybody that close; I wasn't ready to let
go of the hate and the fear, to open myself to another person,
and to help that person open himself to me.

Now that Rick was gone, I could binge again. I could experience the food, develop a relationship to the food, make love
to the food, instead of experiencing Rick, developing a relationship with Rick, making love with Rick. The night we broke
up, I binged. With the food anchored in my belly, I stopped
crying: the food had dried my mouth, my eyes, my emotions.

Six months later, I began another burst of exploration. My
friend Rachel, who was working on documentaries in New
York, invited me to a "rave"—a massive event featuring com-
puter-generated music with a fast beat, young people, and psy-
chedelic drugs, especially MDMA, which is also known as

ecstasy or X. At this rave, which was in a yawning Manhattan concert hall, I would try an illegal drug for the first time. Ecstasy is a drug that affects serotonin levels for three to five hours. Serotonin is a neurotransmitter—a type of brain chemical—that regulates mood and appetite, among its other functions. Most of the newer antidepressants work by altering serotonin levels. Ecstasy works by flooding a person's body with serotonin, making her/him feel empathetic, open, and caring.

Ecstasy has been legally used in psychotherapy in Switzerland. In the presence of a trained therapist, a patient takes a dose of ecstasy and discusses issues she/he has been afraid to confront. Potential issues include the fear, guilt, and sadness among cancer patients; physical or sexual abuse inflicted in the past or present; problems in relationships with parents, spouses, friends, children. Some of those Swiss patients were bulimic.

I am very aware of the dangers of drugs—whether the drug is nicotine or alcohol or ecstasy. I am also aware, from my eating disorder, of other important factors: many substances can be addictive, including food; there's a difference between substance use and substance abuse, whatever the substance; different substances entail different risks, which must be recognized, considered, and respected; some serious problems are inherent in all substances, while others arise from improper use of the substance; and there are some benefits to almost all substances—for example, chocolate and sugar can give pleasure, alcohol can be relaxing, marijuana can ease the effects of glaucoma. Ecstasy can be used relatively safely if a person takes it in moderation and follows the proper precautions. So can alcohol. So can food. Ecstasy can be abused if a person takes too much at one time, takes it often, or thinks the drug is the answer for finding happiness or relief.

At the rave, people were all around me—people in groups, people shifting past one another, people smiling, people talk-

ing. Bottles of water were being sold. Computers displayed psy-
chedelic colors and shapes. Huge screens flashed movement,
color, and form. Rachel's tall figure walked through the scene
with a sense of knowing confidence—she had been to raves and
tried ecstasy before—but also with a sense of wonder at all the
stimuli around her.

After a final moment of consideration, Rachel and I each
took 60 milligrams of ecstasy. As I swallowed the capsule, my
hands shook. What was I putting in my body? Would I be per-
manently affected? Would I hurt myself? Soon I stopped asking
myself those questions. Soon the music filled me. Rachel said
she was dancing with the lights, and she was. My arms floated
high above my body; my hands were fascinating, beautiful.
They circled to create form from movement, they captured the
music. My hands lowered, touched my hips. This is my body.
My body is not an outline, not a number on a scale. My
body is not the size of my pants or the bulge in my belly. My body
has power, it has substance, it is form and movement. My
body is beauty. My body can move its shoulders and hips to the
music that enters me. It can whisper to other people that I love
them, that I care for them. My body has its own needs, its own
desires—to be treated well, to be fed well, to exercise and move
and dance; to hug someone, to give someone comfort, and to
spread itself in sexual joy.

That night, among thousands of people dancing, talking, sitting, hugging, my body was not my adversary, it was a part of me
that gave me strength. It was a part of me that I could embrace.
That night, I connected with, listened to, and loved my body. I
experienced a feeling I had never before known.

The comedown from ecstasy was rough. The next day I felt
tired, my muscles ached. Two days later I felt a bit sad, because
my serotonin level had been depleted on the ecstasy trip. By the
third day I was back to normal. But I was never the same. I had
experienced that previously unknown feeling of connection

with my body and my sense of compassion. Once I knew that feeling, I knew what was possible, what I could work for. I understood. I felt. Some people reach that feeling for the first time when they walk on a beach alone or swim in the water with the sun and sea licking their body. I reached that feeling when I took ecstasy. In order to be true to my experience, I decided to include this story in my book, even though it might be controversial.

I don't think people should automatically go out and use ecstasy or any other drug, legal or illegal. Drugs are potent substances that must be treated with respect. People who use drugs must respect their body and mind enough to know their limits. Those with eating disorders are highly susceptible to alcohol abuse; they are apt to transfer their need for relief in food to a need for relief in alcohol. Therefore everyone, especially people with eating disorders or depressive and anxiety disorders, must be aware and careful when using any substance. I wasn't ready to drink alcohol, let alone take ecstasy, until after I graduated from college. Before that I was too focused on my need for a release.

But I also know that drugs don't always have negative consequences, depending on the drug, the person's mind-set, and the setting in which the drug is taken. *Drug, set, and setting.* Eating a piece of cake with friends is different from eating a whole cake by oneself. Drinking a cocktail with friends is different from drinking a bottle of Jack Daniel's by oneself. Taking ecstasy occasionally to experience the feeling is different from thinking a drug is a savior from depression. Drug, set, and setting.*

My ecstasy excursion didn't enable me to flush away my eating disorder. I started bingeing again a week after the rave as a

*Sociologist Norman Zinberg developed this concept. For a more in-depth discussion of it, see Norman E. Zinberg, *Drug, Set, and Setting* (New Haven: Yale University Press, 1984).

way to cope with work, stress, and sadness. As I had done for the last eight years, I hated my body, feared my body, and ignored its needs. But still, that night of the rave I had an experience that helped me move forward along my path—a path that eventually led to the ability to let go of my eating disorder.

Due to my job, colleagues, writing, and exploration, my eating disorder became less intense during August and September. Instead of drowning my emotions by means of the eating disorder, I often let myself find an equilibrium—find where my body and spirit wanted to go without my mind telling me I couldn't go there.

My body and spirit didn't want to walk into a gym again. I had worked out in a gym seven days a week, one and a half hours each day, for five years, missing maybe ten days a year. Exercising that hard was part of the eating disorder. I had burned the calories, worked the body, pushed the body, manipulated the body. I had compared myself with other women in the gym—those strong, thin women in their designer bodysuits with the single slit of fabric up their little round behinds. I had told myself that the exercising was the only thing that prevented me from becoming a sloth: *Even if I don't look good in a bathing suit, even if I have a gut, even if I binge, I am athletic. I'm not fat and lazy. Damnit, I am athletic.*

Since I wasn't going to the gym anymore but I wanted to exercise my body, I joined an Afro-Brazilian dance class. At my fourth class, I thoroughly got into the "zone"—that place where time, space, emotion, and thought are suspended and the body lets itself move, express, and feel. My arms flung outward and my head waved side to side. The drums were fast and hard; they drove my body. I didn't care about the other people in class, I didn't care about how I looked, I just accepted the music into my body and danced. I was free. My body was free.

Later that month I looked up "belly dancing" in the phone book. When I went to my first class that same day, I immediately connected with the belly-dancing moves, music, and feel-ing. Belly dancing, which is a dance only for women, cherish-es the curves of a woman's body, the softness of her arms, the roundness of her breasts and belly. It celebrates the parts of the body I wanted to cut off. Those belly-dancing lessons helped me accept my body and feel its power. Like my ecstasy trip, it didn't put an end to the eating disorder, but it helped me expe-rience my body, my surroundings, and myself in a different way. Those experiences would build, moving me forward and helping me let go.

The next step in moving forward was a two-week vacation to Amsterdam in September. The first few days of the trip, I rent-ed a bike and rode through the city, turning down random streets, stopping when I saw or felt something that urged me to do so. As I biked through some little towns outside Amsterdam one afternoon, the dark sky started raining. I stopped the bike and stood in the rain; after a moment of stillness, I waved my head side to side and let the thick wetness of my hair hit my face. On this trip to Amsterdam, I didn't need to binge to get out of my head and into my body; I could do it by going to a museum, biking alone, meeting new people, observing others, letting nature touch me and wash me.

That night I met Arno, a friend of a colleague of mine in New York. Arno is a Dutch researcher and writer on psyche-delics. Sitting close to him on his couch, I told him about my biking excursion in the rain, about a sculpture I had seen in a museum of an Indian goddess, her hands expressive, strong, and sensual. I told him that when I had looked at the stone of that sculpture, I could feel her body moving rhythmically, I could sense the connection of her mind and body and spirit. Arno listened. I could see his blue eyes. I could feel his body next to me. I showed him the way the Indian statue's hands were poised. That's when I used my hands—my own expres-sive, strong, sensual hands—and I touched him.

I was exploring. Arno helped me explore. He cooked dinner several nights, and I ate without the consuming fear of getting fat or needing more. That fear was crowded out by so many wonderful feelings. We walked around the city, my private tour guide and I. We went dancing at night. We made love. As I got to know Arno over the next ten days, I learned much about his approach to life. He constantly explored, and he wasn't one to commit. I felt free with his freedom; I needed that freedom at that point in my life. I needed to feel with a man who felt much, and felt it strongly, and then left the feeling for the next one.

FEELING ISN'T ALWAYS pleasant. Part of giving up my eating disorder meant feeling the highs, and part meant feeling the lows.

Each time I explored—each time I opened myself to new people and experiences—I weakened the ability of my eating disorder to keep me safe and numb. I did so even though I didn't yet know healthy ways of dealing with the emotions and situations I now faced—emotions and situations I had suppressed and avoided through my eating disorder for almost a decade. At this point, my body didn't know how to experience sadness or jealousy or loss without turning inward and temporarily shutting off.

It was wet, the air was moist, the sidewalk damp. My face was downturned and lifeless, my body was raw meat. Someone could have cut back and forth through my body, back and forth with a sharp knife, and I would have felt nothing. This is depression—this feeling that nothing is important, that I have left my body, that my mind is dull and thoughts don't form, that my spirit is dead.

I could see people watching me as I walked on 101st and Broadway. Some seemed concerned, others disgusted by this zombie they observed. I didn't care about them, about their concern or disgust toward me. Their opinions didn't matter.

Nothing mattered. Would my next step be into a moving car? I didn't care. It might or it might not. It didn't matter. Nothing mattered. It took too much energy for something to matter. I didn't have the energy. There was no energy. Living, dying. Nothing mattered.

Before Amsterdam, I wouldn't have let my emotions sink so deep into fully felt depression. I would have generated a frenzy of thoughts and actions around food, and then I would have binged and purged to shut down my emotions. But in the month after Amsterdam, the eating disorder was inadequate to hide this void of depression. I now felt a complete loss of my coping mechanism: I had no urge to binge. None. Food was not soothing to me. My mouth and stomach rejected it. Instead I felt waves of depression. I wanted a break from living, a break from obligations. Every obligation became momentous, whether it was meeting a work deadline and paying my bills, or getting out of bed and finding a clean towel.

I'm not sure how long I had been walking when my head turned right and I saw a pay phone. I moved to the phone and called a friend. That took energy and effort. That was an assertion of life. As I cried into the phone, my emotions flowed again. I discovered that I could let my emotions sink into me without smothering them with food, and I would live through it.

With this new maturity, I went to Los Angeles for a drug policy reform conference. Before the meetings began, I took a walk on the beach and thought about letting my mind think and my body feel, about connecting the mind, body, and spirit. I imagined that the three could work together: one might emerge in any given situation and later fade back into balance; then another might emerge in a different situation. I thought of the lack of balance in my life, the way I let my mind almost constantly dominate, the way my body reacted against that dominance with violence—the violence of trying to assert itself through bingeing or one-night stands. I thought of the beauty I'd felt when the three were more in balance and my body emerged in a positive sense, as it did when I was dancing; or my mind emerged in a positive sense, as it did when I wrote a good article at work; or my spirit emerged in a positive sense, as it did when I first kissed Rick. Those times when I achieved a balance were the times I escaped the "all or none."

In this contemplative mood I went to the morning's plenary session, where I heard a speaker with passion in his voice. He was talking about drug education, about a study he had conducted showing that current "Just Say No" programs were ineffective and counterproductive. I met Josh the next day at a small gathering of friends. We talked about his work, my eating disorder, relationships, making ourselves vulnerable in order to grow. We slept with each other that night, knowing he would be leaving for his home in Berkeley the next day while I would be flying back to Manhattan.

As he drove me to the airport, we both felt a connection we weren't ready to lose. From across the country, our relationship grew. My intuition told me we could care for and learn with each other, and I trusted that intuition.

Each night we talked on the phone and revealed new things; each day I worked at my job with increasing frustration; each evening I worked on my book *Inner Hunger* with increasing sadness. Nothing seemed to fit: not the job, not the book, not the boyfriend who lived three thousand miles away. After going through August and September without much of an urge to binge, I began to binge and purge daily. Food again became a comfort. The depression fell away, and the bulimia reemerged from its hibernation. Its ability to help me cope was weakening—I could feel it weakening—but I didn't know any other way to keep myself going to work, writing the book, and making myself open with a man.

*I'm such a hypocrite. You fucking hypocrite! How can you*

*help other people when you can't even help yourself!* My skull echoed with the sounds of my internal screams. *You hypocritical bitch! How can you help other people get rid of their eating disorders when you can't even get rid of your own?* I was pacing in my little box apartment. *I can't do it anymore. I need to get out of here.* My computer screen was glowing with the text of my manuscript, sneering at me as I stood with vomit on my breath and food wrappers at my feet.

The phone rang. I knew it was Josh before I picked it up. As we talked, I started crying. "I can't take it anymore! I binged today, Josh. I didn't want to, but I did it. I feel gross. How could I do it? I'm writing the book and I thought I was over it. How could I do it again?" For the first time I expressed my fear and frustration about my eating disorder when I was feeling that fear and frustration. For the first time I trusted someone else and I trusted myself.

Josh wasn't shocked. He didn't think I was gross. He listened and comforted. After a while, he said softly, with his caring voice, "You have a choice."

The voices in my head started screaming again. *Bullshit! Don't tell me I have a choice! Don't you think I want to stop?! Don't you think I try?! I don't want to feel this anymore, do you think I choose to feel this?* "I don't think it's as easy as that, Josh." My voice was cold, and Josh heard it.

"I don't mean that it's easy to stop. I mean that you can take responsibility for your actions, without judging yourself. Without judging yourself, okay?" He meant that if I felt the need to binge, I could binge. For over nine years, the eating disorder had been an effective coping mechanism: I'd been strong enough to discover and live with my eating disorder. Therefore I didn't have to judge myself harshly because I binged. But I did need to become aware that I was making a decision each time I binged. Nothing was making me binge, I needed to binge. Acknowledge that, accept that. Then you can change it.

Josh and I talked for another hour on the phone, and the

next day red roses were delivered to my apartment. Josh and I had shared that night. I had made myself vulnerable to him, and he had accepted that trust with the caring it required. Since he wasn't in New York to hold me, he sent me roses. I rubbed the sweet petals on my face and let them caress my cheek and forehead and lips.

After visiting Josh in California, I decided to move west. It was a risk for both of us. But I had nothing to keep me in New York, and I had something and someone to explore in California. I found someone to take over my lease in New York and I signed a six-month contract to work from a home office for the drug policy research institute. I would move in January. He would fly to New York, and we would drive cross-country to our Berkeley home.

Good. Fine. Great. *What the hell am I doing! I'm moving into the house of a man I've known for less than a month. I'm giving up my own space. I'm going cross-country for a man?! But I'm a feminist! Am I compromising myself to be with a man? How can I do this?* The bulimia intensified during the month before the move because I needed to cope with the fear of establishing a relationship and the fear of changing my life in such an abrupt and complete way. The bulimia also intensified because I thought I would have to give up my eating disorder in January, once I moved in with Josh. After all, we would sleep together each night in the same bed, and I couldn't get into that bed with my belly distended, hurting from food. I had three weeks left to binge and purge, then I would have to kill my bulimia.

The three weeks were up. On our drive cross-country, Josh and I strolled in the sun of Charleston, got serenaded by a blues singer in New Orleans, walked on the white sands of New Mexico. I opened myself more and more to him and felt his spirit entering me more deeply. As I felt myself love Josh more, I made myself eat less. I was trying to lose weight to look good for him and to be in control for myself. By the time we got to Berkeley, I was starved. I didn't go to bed with him that first night. I stayed up, telling him I wanted to read, and ate half a box of cookies. I did the same the next night. And the third night. I needed to eat. I was holding tight to my relationship with food, afraid to let it go and to pursue my relationship with Josh.

I needed to eat to help me numb out and feel safe in my new home, but I also recognized that the eating disorder and my inability to talk about it with Josh were hurting the relationship.

"Josh, I feel sad," I told him as we were lying in bed, two weeks after our arrival in Berkeley. "I've been bingeing and throwing up a lot."

"I know."

My stomach muscles contracted, trying to suppress the embarrassment that had started to grow. "You know?"

"Yeah, but I thought you'd tell me when you were ready. And you did." His words contained no anger. But they were firm. "So what do you want to do about this, Marianne?"

"I think I should start seeing a therapist again."

He nodded his head and spoke low and soft. "You can do it. You're strong."

The next day I called a therapist recommended by an old friend of Josh's. I talked with Amy on the phone for a while. Even over the phone line, I liked the feeling I got from her. I made an appointment for that week.

Halfway through the first session, I knew I would continue with Amy until I had traveled far in the process of giving up my eating disorder. She was young, professional yet compassionate, interested in what I was saying. She didn't allow long awkward pauses, because I could make the most progress if I felt comfortable. She didn't ask global questions about my life, for example: "So, Marianne, tell me about your upbringing. . . ." She knew that the major issues and important details of my past would emerge in time. In the beginning, she wanted to know what I was feeling and doing right now, here in Berkeley, California.

Over the next year and a half, I came to appreciate Amy's style. She explored my past with me as a way to understand the sources of my current thoughts, feelings, and behaviors, and as a way to bring closure. But she also realized that revisiting the past and understanding root causes are only two components of any attempt to make changes in one's life. We also had to talk about today, now, tomorrow. "What are you going to do when you leave the session to try to listen to your body?" or "How about if you try eating a cookie in a café rather than eating it fast in the car before you get home? How would that feel different? Do you think you can try that?" or "How does Josh's reaction feel to you? Where do you feel it? How else can you respond to him so you communicate your feelings?" When I left the sessions with Amy, I felt I had either gained a greater understanding of myself or determined a clear strategy to approach the experiences I would be facing in the next few days. Often I left feeling I had achieved both. Until I worked with Amy, I didn't realize that these skills were what I wanted and needed from a therapist.

But even though I felt good about my new relationship with Amy, I'd had enough therapy to know that my eating disorder wouldn't disappear immediately. That realization was made all the more clear when Josh took a short business trip to Southern California. I planned the binge for days before he left: what I would eat, where I would buy what I would eat, when I would buy what I would eat. I felt excitement and fear at the knowledge that no one would be around to stop me from bingeing. I told Amy about my strong desire to binge, I told her I adamantly wanted to do it despite my fear of the consequences. "Okay, then I'm not going to try to stop you. If you need to binge this week, then you can binge. What I want to work on is taking some of the judgment out of it." But I was too frazzled to absorb much of the subsequent conversation.

After buying bread, chocolate, muffins, and cookies at various stores, I ate as much as I could until my stomach felt a tremendous pain that was simultaneously sharp and dull. Before I moved to the bathroom to vomit, I put the remaining food in the kitchen sink, turned on the water, and drenched it with dish soap. I wanted to ensure that I wouldn't eat any more, even after I'd vomited and created more room in my stomach for food.

When I was done throwing up, I paced through the apartment fast, heart beating fast, hands moving fast—through my hair, clasped behind my head, through my hair again. I walked to the sink and looked at the food, soggy and soapy. "NO! NO! No, no, no!" I wanted to eat the food. How could I have destroyed the food? My hand reached into the sink and lifted the bread and cookies from the soapy water. "NO!" I squeezed them and felt the food ooze through my hands, the consistency of vomit. "No, no, I want that food, why did I ruin that food, no, no, no, no, no, no, no. . . . I NEED IT, I NEED THAT FOOD!"

I knew I was losing control. I forced my body onto the floor and pounded my hand on the concrete foundation. I could feel my hand sting. I wanted to hurt my body. I got up from the kitchen floor, moved to the wall in the bathroom, and banged with my fist. High-pitched buzzing screamed in my ears. I fell to the floor in the living room, too exhausted to stand. I felt the dead gums of my mouth, charred by the acid of my vomit. I panted until my breath became more smooth and slow. I picked up the phone, dialed mechanically, and let the phone ring until I heard an answering machine. "Amy, it's Marianne Apostolides. Um, can you call me back?" She did. I saw her that afternoon.

"I don't want to alarm you, Marianne, but you are in crisis."

*Great.* "What I mean by that is that your coping mechanisms don't work anymore. The bingeing and purging aren't giving you what you need anymore. So what we're going to work on is developing new coping mechanisms, and trying to build your sense of self so your need for coping mechanisms changes." I was sitting on Amy's green couch, curled tight in the left-hand corner for protection. She was right, I was in crisis. I felt like a helpless kid looking up to an adult, tears on my face, asking for her to give me strength, asking her to make it okay. Later I learned that Amy couldn't give me strength or make it okay; only I could do those things. But Amy could help me find my strength, and she could help me find different paths for creating change.

I purged only a handful of times after that big binge/purge and the panic attack that followed. The purging was getting too hard for me physically and emotionally. Right after I threw up, I would move around, unable to sit still; I would become frazzled and hyper. After the initial hysteria wore off, I would cry and sink into self-criticism.

Soon my body started resisting the walk to the bathroom to purge: my mouth, hand, stomach, and throat didn't want to go. They were repelled. For months, my mind had known that purging was too hurtful, and now my body had learned. I was able to heed my body's pleas because I was working both in and out of therapy to find new ways of dealing with my emotions, because my body physically couldn't take the trauma anymore, and because I had the support of Josh. The last purge wasn't an elaborately planned big "hooray" as I had anticipated it would be; instead it was a small binge and purge that left me feeling silly. Not angry or judgmental, just silly because my body and mind knew I didn't need it anymore.

Even though I let go of the purging, I couldn't let go of my need for relief in food. But since I was no longer purging, my body could no longer incorporate massive amounts of food at one sitting—it could no longer binge. So I started eating bits of food in secret: two pieces of bread while Josh was in the shower, a handful of chips and some cereal while Josh was jogging, chocolates when I was cleaning up the kitchen after dinner. Any opportunity to eat some food in secret triggered a response in me: *Do it, Mare, do it now while you have the chance. Eat it!* I ate more than felt good, ate when I couldn't be seen by people who knew me, ate with a certain desperation, and felt guilt after eating. I labeled this uncontrolled eating of smaller amounts of food "grazing," and many in the psychological community call it "compulsive eating." Compulsive eating is a sister behavior to anorexia and bulimia: all three are frightening and consuming, all three are coping mechanisms for deep psychological issues, and all three prevent a person from doing everything she feels she wants to do.

Amy and I discussed the fact that the compulsive eating was a phase that I would have to go through as I moved away from the bulimia. In this phase, my body felt better than it had when I binged; my mind felt I was making progress. But I was impatient: I wanted to be done with my food issues completely, I didn't want to feel restricted because of my anxieties about food and body.

Over the next few months of impatience and compulsive eating, I learned that I would have to accept the whole process of giving up my eating disorder, no matter how long that process took.

# E I G H T

■

# Letting Go

VEN as I was letting go of the eating disorder, it was affecting me as a woman, as a worker, as a member of a couple. It was also affecting Josh—his sense of self, his emotions, his ability to relax and explore in the relationship. I never understood the power of the eating disorder's reverberations until Josh let his tension turn to anger one night.

Nothing grabbed my interest in the organic foods grocery store that night, so I decided to go home and make myself a baked potato with some vegetables, cheese, and beans. I was proud of myself: instead of taking whatever I saw at the market, I paused to consider what my body wanted to eat. But Josh hadn't spoken since we left the store, and I sensed a tension inside him. While driving home, I interrupted the silence with the question "Are you mad at me?"

"Yes! Yes, I'm mad at you!" His words bounced around the car. "We go to the organic foods store because you say you want

something from there. And then you take twenty minutes looking around. And then you don't get anything. So now I'm left
wondering, Is she gonna get upset because she didn't get food?
Is she gonna start to cry? Is she gonna binge tonight? What can
I do to make sure she doesn't binge?" Josh and I were both
panting now, Josh in anger, me in shock. I hadn't realized that
over the last few months, my spinning emotions were like a tornado that sucked Josh's emotions into the whirl. When we got
home that night, we began an ongoing dialogue about the way
my eating disorder affected us as a couple.

Through our new dialogue, I learned that my daily crying
was hurting Josh and his sense of self. Each day he saw me
upset, wanted to help, and felt powerless to do anything. Even
though he knew that he wasn't responsible for making me
happy, he thought he should at least be able to make me less
sad; if he couldn't, he felt he was failing as a partner. But it
wasn't just the sadness that bothered Josh, it was the rapidity of
the mood swings and the changes in body image. I could be
laughing and goofy at 6 P.M., but by 7:30 I'd be crying, hiding
under the covers, making nasty comments. On any given night,
Josh didn't know if I would feel sensual and sexual, or if I would
be disgusted by my body and fearful of touch. That made him
feel less comfortable with me, less able to love my body.
Without knowing it, I was stifling the mutual passion and ease
that partners seek to develop.

Because of my zigzagging emotions, Josh felt as if he had to
walk on eggshells when dealing with me. He wondered if I
would get offended when he innocently said, "Are you exercising today?" or "Isabella Rossellini is electric on screen." When
my sense of self was low, I attached a charge to Josh's state-
ments: when he said, "Are you exercising today?" I heard, "You
really should exercise today, because you're starting to get flabby and you're eating a lot, so you'd really better exercise." When
he said, "Isabella Rossellini is electric," I heard, "There are so

many beautiful women, more beautiful than you, and I would gladly be with them instead of you because they're so gorgeous."

The day after Josh and I first discussed his feelings about my eating disorder, I spent an entire session with Amy talking about the effects of my bulimia on the relationship. "It sounds like you're struggling with the whole issue of being your own container," she commented. I didn't understand. Amy saw the confusion in my face. "What I mean is that sometimes you don't contain your emotions inside you. You used to act them out or shove them down through eating. Now you get very withdrawn or angry or even nasty." Now this discussion sounded familiar. Theresa, the first therapist I went to, called this "sitting with feelings." Amy explained that we could work together to help me learn how to contain my emotions—how to hold them inside me and explore what I feel.

"I see your face looks skeptical, Marianne. What are you thinking?"

"I'm thinking that it sounds hard."

"It is hard. I don't want to say to you, 'Contain your emotions,' without recognizing the difficulty of doing that, and without helping you through it." She paused, checking to see if I was absorbing her words. "And I also want to recognize that containing your emotions can be scary. I mean, why would you want to feel your emotions when you've developed a whole system—a really well-designed system—to shut them down?"

"Because shutting them down doesn't work anymore. Because it hurts me too much and it hurts my relationship too much." Amy was nodding her head. But I wasn't sure I could do it. I wasn't sure I was capable of holding my emotions inside me.

Amy saw my discomfort, and began to outline the first step I could take in learning to be my own container. That step was to let therapy be my container: with Amy I could let my emotions emerge, and together we could discuss them, hold them, and deal with my response. This concept of being able to use a therapist to hold emotions during a session is often called the "therapeutic container." Amy explained that a person can begin to experience the sensation of containing emotions when she holds them with the help of a therapist. She may feel a nervous energy rise in her, her muscles may tense up, she may want to yell at her parents or her boss or the man who raped her. If that person uses therapy to discuss these feelings, to hold them until they pass, or to determine healthy ways to act on them, she can eventually become her own container. As such, she can move through the day feeling a range and cycle of emotions and experiences without crushing them.

This process is gradual. It was almost a year before I began to contain my own emotions as a natural part of my life. In the interim, I could feel when I was being my own container, and when I was suppressing my emotions because my body and spirit couldn't hold them. And I could always feel secure in the knowledge that I had my therapeutic container once a week and, for several months, twice a week.

Lasting change comes when a client can use the therapeutic container to get beyond crises and experiment with new patterns of thinking, feeling, and acting. Amy and I were slowly realizing that the waves of crises were coming too fast for me, making me focus on being able to breathe rather than learning how to swim.

As I struggled to breathe, I became the "human nighttime tornado"—I tossed and turned at night, unable to give my mind and body a rest. Josh would hug me close in the morning, when our bodies were still soft and warm from sleep. He would tell me about the way I had sobbed during the night, or had made pained noises, or had banged my head against the pillow. During the day, the waves pounded my conscious mind. Little pictures would flash fast through my brain: pictures of my head on the pavement being crushed by a truck, pictures of a gun pointed to my temple and exploding, pictures of my head hitting a wall and cracking with each strike. When the anxiety became overwhelming, I would enter a phase of surrender—I would feel as if my body were floating as it slowly died underwater. My mind would slow, my body would slow, and I would yearn for a release from living.

I told Amy about these feelings. She understood that I was moving through cycles of anxiety and depression. That afternoon she asked if I had ever considered taking an antidepressant. She explained that she didn't think the medication was right for everyone, or that it was a therapist's role to push a client to take an antidepressant. But she encouraged me to think about it, to talk about it with people I trusted, and to talk about it with her when I felt ready.

Antidepressant drugs are a group of medicines that act on brain chemicals called neurotransmitters. The most common group of antidepressants are selective serotonin reuptake inhibitors, or SSRIs. By raising the serotonin level, antidepressants can affect a person's demeanor. In various clinical tests on eating disorders, antidepressants along with talk therapy have had positive outcomes to a greater degree than either talk therapy alone or antidepressants alone.

I was strongly against antidepressants because I thought they would alter my personality—take away who I was, make me dull, dilute my passion. I thought antidepressants meant that I, Marianne, am only a group of chemicals, that my spirit is nothing more than neurotransmitters chasing one another through my brain. I spoke with Josh about antidepressants the night Amy mentioned them. He didn't understand how I could favor the occasional and controlled use of ecstasy or alcohol or other drugs and completely reject antidepressants. They are all drugs on the same continuum, he said. We talked about the fact that an antidepressant, like any other drug, is a tool each person can use to shape her own reality; that it can help different parts of her personality emerge if used properly; and that it can be dangerous both physically and psychologically if used improperly. The day after this conversation with Josh, I got a prescription from my doctor in consultation with my therapist.* I knew I had taken a positive step, but I also knew there were many more steps ahead.

Before I began taking the antidepressant, I lurched from one crisis to another. Afterward I still had crises, but I didn't have them all the time. I stopped crying every day, I stopped hiding under the covers every day, I stopped craving the night so I could sleep. Now that I wasn't constantly overwhelmed, I could concentrate on making substantial changes. I could reexamine my patterns, work with Amy to find different ways to change those patterns, and start to implement those changes in my life. After I stopped bingeing and purging and before I started taking the antidepressant, my focus was often on achieving and maintaining composure so I could work and survive and communicate. Now my focus was on becoming healthy and balanced.

The antidepressant wasn't a cure-all. I don't think it would have been much help if I hadn't been working with a good therapist. And the antidepressant had side effects: it made me sleepy, and it sometimes bothered my stomach, making me feel nauseous right before I ate. But I endured these side effects because the benefits outweighed the annoyances, and because I knew I was only using the medication temporarily, until I had established more healthy patterns.

WITH THE SUBTLE but noticeable help of the antidepressant, I was able to enter a phase in which the eating disorder faded as a presence in my life. The process entailed time, an acceptance of cycles and slipups, and a changed lifestyle. I had to work on

*Most people get an antidepressant prescription from a psychiatrist in consultation with their primary therapist rather than from a doctor in consultation with their primary therapist.

bringing closure to issues from my past, changing habitual behavior patterns, establishing a healthy relationship with my body, developing compassion, and trusting myself as my own container and source of strength. Now that I have progressed into the new phase, I can finish this part of my journey, and finish this story that you have let me share with you.

Amy and I began discussing my past in an in-depth way for the first time since I'd started therapy eight months earlier. We didn't purposely approach the topic; my words simply led us there. "I would push my mother, I would almost dare her to tell me to stop or put me in my place, and she wouldn't. She would yell at me and then I would spit at her . . . and after hours of this we'd finally make up with all this crying and hugging. . . ." My voice started to shake with sadness and embarrassment.

After asking me some questions and listening to my responses, Amy began to understand the dynamic that had existed between my mother and me. I was feeding off my mother's unhappiness, and she was feeding off mine. My mother felt like a failure because she was incapable of keeping both her children healthy and happy. She started to doubt the choices she'd made in her life—mainly the choice to stay home and raise children. She started to wonder what she had achieved when her only daughter was so angry and self-destructive. With that self-doubt and the onset of menopause, my mother needed to channel her own unhappiness, and she channeled it toward me. I accepted that unhappiness and gave her my own sadness in the form of anger—yelling, spitting at her, telling her I would never make the same dumb choices she'd made. We each transferred our unhappiness onto the other. By doing so, we could suppress our emotions and avoid taking the difficult step of working through our problems.

"Where was your father while all this was happening between you and your mom?"

"He was working," I responded. "I mean, sometimes he

broke up arguments between my mother and me, but usually he was out of the picture."

Amy smiled. "We can't let him off the hook that easily! I don't want to blame either of your parents, but I want to explore the whole family dynamic." Amy and I had previously discussed my father's obsessive behavior, but only now did I start to understand that his absence as an emotional support had allowed the eating disorder to develop and grow for ten years.

After we discussed the family dynamic, Amy put a name to it. "There's something called the IP, which means the 'identified patient.' Usually there's one person in a family who manifests the family's problems, and that's the IP." Although everyone in the family has problems, the IP is the one who allows those problems to surface in her/his behavior.

Children can sense parental unhappiness, financial strain, drinking problems, etc.; when they absorb such tension without knowing how to process it, they often seek a release in a variety of destructive and self-destructive behaviors. That relieves other family members from the burden of examining their own issues, because they can instead focus on the IP. In my case, I sensed my father's obsessiveness and discomfort with emotions, and my mother's low self-confidence. I took on their tension, added it to my own, and manifested it through my eating disorder.

"Marianne, how do you feel about being the IP in the family?"

"I feel pissed at my parents. Why should I have to go through all of this? Why should I feel guilty and stick my finger down my throat? I mean, why did I have to take on all their problems?"

"It makes sense to be angry. It was hard on you," Amy agreed sympathetically.

"But I don't want to feel like I'm a victim, because my parents would never deliberately hurt me. . . . I just don't want to blame them."

"I agree. It's not about blame. But I also don't want you to blame yourself, which you seem to do a lot. You put a judgment on yourself about how bad you were for having an eating disorder. But you're not bad. You were acting in a way to protect yourself and deal with your environment in the best way you knew how."

Before I left that day, Amy said that we would use the next few sessions to work on bringing closure to the unhealthy relationships I had had with my parents in the past, and on developing practical ways my parents and I could move forward in our relationship.

The next week Amy and I did mild hypnotherapy, which some therapists call "active imagination." Amy suggested we try this technique because it can help a patient tap into deep feelings without the interference of her mind. I was a bit nervous about hypnotherapy, but I trusted Amy and I wanted to make progress in the work we were doing together.

I laid on a blanket on the floor, closed my eyes, and began to breathe deeply. Amy lowered the lights and softened her voice. "Your breathing is even and smooth. With each breath out, you're more relaxed. You can feel the tension leaving your body." Once I was deeper into that hypnotic trance, Amy said I would soon find myself in a room, and that I should tell her when I got there. After searching through a dark hallway in my mind, I felt myself in the kitchen of my parents' house. I was sixteen. Amy asked if anyone was in the room with me. I looked around at the Wedgwood-blue kitchen cabinets, the half-opened window, and the olive green oven. "Yes. My mom is in the room. At the other corner of the room near the oven. And our dog is there, too."

"What's happening, Marianne?"

I waited for the action, the movement of my mother and me

and the dog. "It's very noisy. We're yelling. The dog is scared. She's next to me shaking. She hates it when we fight."

"What are you saying?"

I listened, but I didn't hear anything for a long time. Then my eyes and ears focused. "My arms are clasped around my head. And I'm yelling. *'Make it stop. There's too much in my head, it's too fast. I can't feel it anymore, it's too much. Mom, please make it stop.'* "

"Let yourself feel that for a minute, Marianne." Amy became silent. I felt tears on my face. "Marianne, you're now going to leave the kitchen and walk into a big open field. You can tell me when you get there."

I felt myself moving. The dog was with me. "I'm here."

"What do you feel?"

"I can breathe again. It's very open, I feel very open. I'm playing with the dog. . . . That feels nice."

"That's great, Marianne. You can hold on to that feeling for a minute." Amy was again silent, letting me remain in the peaceful moment. "Now, Marianne, soon we're going to come back to this room. But before we do, I want you to let go of all that extra information in your head. Let it float out of you into that big, open field. Any information you need, you will keep. But the rest can flow out of you. Let it flow right out."

I felt my muscles relax as I let myself release the "extra information."

"Now you are becoming more aware of your breathing. You can feel the temperature in this room. You can hear the sounds of this room right now. And when you're ready, you can open your eyes and join me here."

"Wow." That's all I could say. I felt a bit groggy, but also energized by the hypnotherapy's power.

"That was wonderful. How did it feel?" Amy was smiling as she spoke.

"The letting go of information was scary, because I wanted to keep it in my head. But as you were talking I started feeling like I keep too much in my head, and I want to let go of some thoughts and iterations in there."

"How about when you were in the kitchen?"

"I felt like I wasn't yelling at my mother or mad at her or anything. I was yelling because there was so much inside my head, and it was all overwhelming. All I could do was yell. That's the only way I could stop my head from spinning." Amy nodded. Our session was over, but I went home thinking about that trance.

Through the active imagination, I gained a greater understanding of my relationship with my mother. When I yelled at her, I wasn't angry with her, I was frightened by the rushing thoughts inside my mind. I was yelling because I didn't know how else to ask for help. And I realized that my mother didn't know how else to help me except to submit to the anger: she didn't know how to help me get into the metaphoric open field and release the extra information. And so we remained trapped in our dynamic of sadness.

Because of my work with Amy, I felt comfortable talking with my mother about our past. I started the discussion on one of our trips to Lenox, Massachusetts, a little town near the Tanglewood Estate that is a mecca for music, theater, and dance each summer. It was raining, not too hard, but enough to make the windshield wipers swing side to side. Soothed by the beating of the rain and the rhythm of the wipers, I slipped into a trancelike state where my mind flowed free without judgment. I thought about the differences among the three trips my mother and I had made to this wooded town. So much had changed. The first year I was just out of college, angry and unstable, nasty toward my mother. We spent whole afternoons in silence as I let my anger create a wall between me and other people, and between me and my deeper emotions.

I remembered the second year, when the trip was less

charged. My mother and I could give each other more space. We spent a lot of time in each other's presence without saying anything; instead of exchanging words, we absorbed the cool summer air and the safe feeling of being together. A week after I returned home from that second trip, I made my big break in self-perception and self-presentation, when I tossed out the makeup and high heels for jeans, and when I quit the gym for belly-dancing lessons.

This was the third year. The rain began to fall harder, drawing me out of my daydream and into the car with my mother. "Mom, I was talking to Amy, and maybe when you come to Berkeley, the two of us can see her and talk about the eating disorder and how you felt and, you know, just to get everything into the open." She didn't say anything. "I want to know how you felt when I was in high school. I'm not mad at you and Dad, but sometimes I feel resentful that you guys didn't talk with me about my eating disorder. I think you should know how I felt and I should know how you felt so we can give some closure to it. . . . Do you know what I mean?"

"Yes." She paused, trying to keep the tears from leaving her throat. "I felt so sad, Marianne. I saw you get so sad, and I never felt that sadness when I was growing up. I never felt that. . . . And you were hurting yourself and being so hard on yourself, and there was nothing I could do! Sometimes I wished you would take it out on me and not be so hard on yourself."

"But I did take it out on you, Mom! I was so mean to you and Dad, but I didn't know how else to be. . . ." After a deep breath, I continued. "But I feel like I want to know how *you* felt. Amy said it's natural for parents to feel angry at their kids who have an eating disorder, not in a bad way, but just because it's really hard on the family."

"No, I never felt anger. I loved you so much, and you were just a little girl hurting yourself. That made me so sad. I wanted to help you so much, and there was nothing I could do."

"But you could've done something, Mom. You could've sat down and talked with me instead of getting upset and yelling at me. We could've talked about it." My voice was gentle, letting my mother know that I wasn't carrying anger at her for not getting me help.

"I went to a psychiatrist a few times and he asked me if you were having trouble at school or putting yourself in physical danger. And I said you weren't, so he said I should leave you alone, and you'd grow out of it."

"That psychiatrist gave you shitty advice." For the first time that night, my voice became hard.

"I'm so sorry." She was crying. Tears were creeping down her face like the rain creeping down the window. "No, no, Mom, it's not your fault. I don't blame you. You and Dad did the best you knew how, I know that." We were both crying, not too hard, but enough to release the energy of our emotions. I felt like my mother and I had reached a new level in our relationship—a level that was possible only when both of us experienced ourselves in a new way: when my mother felt that she was a confident, competent person, and when I experienced a deep love that allowed me to get beyond the scab of anger and toward compassion and understanding.

After my mother and I got back from Lenox, I spent a day at home on Long Island. My father and I took our big white poodle Charlie for a long walk around town. I love seeing my dad around dogs: he opens up, becoming goofy and free in a way I rarely ever see.

On the walk, I started asking my father questions about his life in Greece. In my twenty-four years, I had never really learned what he had experienced as a child, what had shaped him into the man who is my father. As I asked questions, he told me about his childhood for the first time. He told me about living in Nazi-occupied Greece, about the shortages of food, the lack of power. He used to wait in a long line to get the rationed loaf of bread that he would share with the family. Big blocks of ice were brought to the house sporadically to prevent food from spoiling. People who died of starvation in the streets were carted away in garbage trucks. His father was a veterinarian and an important member of the resistance movement that organized against the Nazis and the Greek Communists; he was killed in an ambush. No one knew the details, but there were rumors. The body was never found.

Almost an hour into our walk, my father started playing with the dog, perhaps to escape the feelings my questions had stirred within him. For the rest of the walk, our conversation was lighter. But when we got home, I thought about what my father had said. I could understand how a person who has seen and felt death as a child would cut himself off from certain deep feelings. That protective mechanism didn't mean that my father lacked emotions, but it did mean that he was uncomfortable recognizing those emotions, expressing them, and being aware of them as he felt them. As a way to protect himself from the powerful emotions that were somewhere inside him, my father was obsessive and compulsive. It makes sense that he focused his obsession on food, because he had been forced to focus on food as a child—waiting in line for bread and hoping the ice would come so the food didn't spoil. And it also makes sense that he focused his obsession on the body, because as a boy he had struggled to stay strong and avoid the death and starvation that were all around him.

That afternoon I felt no anger or blame. But I did feel sadness—sadness at the horror my father had experienced as a child, sadness at the fact that I had reacted to him by developing an eating disorder, sadness that we had never before talked about these issues. I also felt a closeness to my father; I felt a pure happiness that our relationship had changed, that we were talking with each other as adults who loved and cared for each other.

As George and I became adults and grew closer to our parents, we also grew apart from each other. After idolizing him for years, I discovered who I was, and I discovered that I would never have chosen for myself the life he is leading. He is a good person, an honest and caring person, but I could never be a business lawyer. And he could never be a freelance writer who feels it is important to write about love and relationships and hurt. Our different paths and priorities have created a strain between us. We are just starting to address that strain, to acknowledge that we want to talk about our past together, our feelings as we grew up, and our present lives. Although we aren't fully comfortable with each other as adults yet, I know that we both want to work on our relationship. That knowledge has brought me a sense of peace.

WHILE I WORKED on bringing closure to the past and changing my present relationships with my family, I also needed to alter my basic eating patterns. Amy suggested that I think about keeping a food journal. She explained that the journal wasn't an assignment or something to be graded, it was a tool for gathering valuable information. By helping me create an awareness of what I ate, the times I ate, and the moods I was in when I ate, the journal could help me change my eating patterns. For example, an increased awareness might encourage me to pause before I grazed: Do I really want to eat this next bowl of cereal, or am I okay without it? Amy and I could also look over the journal and notice broad patterns: for example, it seems that I get anxious for carbohydrates at 3:30 or 4 P.M.; and on the days when I don't have a snack in the afternoon, I tend to graze a lot at night because my hunger hasn't been satisfied.

At first I resisted the idea of keeping a journal, fearing that I would have to start eating only the "right" foods at the "right" times. Amy assured me that I didn't have to start the journal until I felt ready. But she also reminded me that keeping a journal didn't obligate me to change my eating habits right away. "You can think of it as an information-gathering exercise," she said. "You're not sure what you're going to do with the information you get, but you're going to gather it so you can use it when you're ready."

For two more months, I needed to continue the phase of letting myself eat whatever I wanted, whenever I wanted it. I needed to feel how grazing affected my mood, my attitude toward my body, my attitude toward myself. I also needed to understand that nothing was restricting my eating—not my parents, not Josh, not my friends. During the months of grazing, I became aware that only I can restrict my eating. Not in order to deny myself, but in order to act within boundaries that I have created based on what feels good to me, what helps me live the way I want to live.

Once I started the food journal, I realized that I wasn't eating enough protein and I wasn't feeding myself when I got hungry in the afternoon. Those habits kept me craving quick fixes, like big cookies and chocolate bars. As I changed my eating patterns, my cravings changed, too; they became more varied depending on what I was doing and feeling that day. I couldn't always listen to those cravings or follow a new pattern. Sometimes I grazed because I felt agitated and wanted to soothe myself, sometimes I ate a big cookie because I could do so without anyone seeing me. But on the whole, my patterns were changing.

As I took care of my eating patterns in a cognitive way, I needed to take care of my body in a meditative way. The first time I did that was on a camping trip. Since I hadn't lost all the weight I had wanted to lose before the trip, I felt apprehensive about going. But once I got into the woods in Oregon, once I heard the stream running and felt the trees sheltering me, my weight didn't matter. There were no mirrors, no billboards of models, no deadlines. There were my friends and me and nature.

On Saturday, the six of us hiked to a clear pond, which was the origin of the stream near our campsite. Everyone on the trip had been to this pond several times, but no one had gone in because it was freezing cold. Our friend Michael walked several yards away, took off his shirt and shoes, and threatened to jump in. "Hey, Michael, if you go in, I'll go in," I yelled, hoping he'd jump.

I didn't see him dive in the first time, I just heard the splash and the laughter that followed. "It's cold!" He had already scooted out of the water by the time I looked. "Marianne, it's your turn now!" I climbed to Michael's spot, took off my shoes and shirt. "Is it really cold?" I looked at him, eyebrows raised. Michael's deep, smooth voice was reassuring. "Oh yes, it's cold . . . but it feels great." I stood by the water, took off my cut-off shorts and my bra, and I dove in. When my head emerged, I heard everyone laughing. *Cold, cold, cold.* I got to the rock and climbed out. I was laughing, too. The water hugged my skin until the sun soaked it up. My naked body felt alive. That day my body and mind and spirit were all connected at the ice-cold pond off the trail off the campsite off the road in Oregon. That afternoon I realized that I didn't have to lose weight in order to experience myself and my body in a beautiful way.

My first formal effort to reconnect with my body was my decision to start seeing a massage therapist every few weeks. By getting therapeutic massages from a licensed massage therapist, I was taking care of myself and helping my body and mind feel calmer, more centered. Massage helped me respect my body; when I respected my body, I didn't want to hurt it by filling it with food it didn't want, or by depriving it of food it did.

After several massages, I felt the urge to exercise again. I hadn't exercised for months, in part because I had become obsessed with calorie counting and tended to push myself too hard whenever I tried to work out. I had recognized those impulses as unhealthy, and decided to back off. But now, after starting to connect with the muscles of my body through massage, I wanted to exercise—not because exercising would burn calories, but because it would feel good to my body.

Before jumping back into aerobics classes, I tried to feel what form of exercise my body wanted, and I listened when it urged me to walk and take yoga classes. By rejuvenating my body through movement, I soon started to feel the desire for more intense exercise. My body was ready for karate, dance, and swimming—and I gladly gave it those presents.

After a month of healthy eating and exercise, I went through a weekend of heavy grazing. Before letting myself sink back into compulsive eating, I remembered Amy's discussion of compassion: if I could give myself compassion when I fell back into old patterns—if I could consider that I'm a good person who is brave to deal with many difficult issues—I could remove some of the judgment that surrounded my eating behavior. Without that judgment, the eating disorder loses much of its power.

I had been nurturing myself with food for a decade. Through work and support, I had learned to nurture myself in other ways, and had moved forward in the process of letting go. With the slipup over the weekend, I was continuing along in that process: I couldn't advance until I let myself feel the food heavy in my stomach without shutting down my body, and I let my anger about the relapse dissolve into compassion.

As I went back to healthy eating the next week, I realized that compassion extended beyond eating. If I wanted to move through my life without a self-destructive coping mechanism, I needed to give compassion to myself and others. If I didn't, I wouldn't be able to deal with the problems and pressures that come with experiencing a full life. I will probably relapse again. When I do, I will know how to deal with it: with the recognition that relapses are part of the process of letting go, with compassion for myself as I go through this difficult part of the process, and with the knowledge that I can bring myself back to a place of emotional and physical health.

AFTER SEVERAL MONTHS without the eating disorder, I felt a clarity that I had never known while I was in the depths of my anorexia and bulimia. I realized that I needed to explore on my own, as a capable woman who is able to experience life without using a coping mechnism in food. I had never before done that, and I couldn't do it while in a relationship with Josh; I would have been dishonest with myself and with Josh if I denied that realization. So with sadness and grief, we said good-bye to each other as lovers.

I am alone now, with myself and the emotions that come with leaving a path that has been nurturing, and starting on one that promises new smells and tastes and colors. My breath is deep and fast as I realize that this is the first time I am exploring on my own as a woman who trusts herself, feels her strength, and fully experiences her needs and fears and wants; this is the first time I am feeding my inner hunger.

# PART
# FIVE

■

# I'm Free

The power of this book and my words is limited. I cannot and do not want to assume the role of a therapist. This book, like any other, is inadequate for treating an eating disorder. But a book can be a useful tool, not only in helping people understand the experience of an eating disorder, but also in providing substantive information that readers can use as they seek further help. In previous chapters, I have tried to help you understand the experience of an eating disorder. In these last chapters, I am try-ing to provide you with information you can use — information based on research articles, books, and consultation with professionals. I don't have the solution to people's eating disorders. But I have my own experience, and a sense of connection with others living in similar unspoken fury.

I have broken this section into three chapters: advice to communities and institutions, advice to people who care about those with eating disorders, and advice to girls and women with eating disorders. In each chapter, I directly address the people to whom I'm giving advice. But I encourage everyone to read the three chapters so we can all understand one another's options and roles in the process of letting go.

# N I N E

■

# Advice to Communities

# and Institutions

LTHOUGH a person cannot release herself from an eating disorder by blaming society, society does contribute to the development of eating disorders, and can contribute to their reduction. People who care about the well-being of girls and women can take specific steps to reform our social institutions. By working to change ourselves and society, we can help those closest to us, and those we have never met.

Everyone in our family and community systems can make a priority of listening to young people, talking with them, and fostering their self-discovered interests. If adults interact with young people in a way that encourages the three "conditions of empowerment"—caring relationships, high expectations, and opportunities for participation—kids can begin to form a healthy sense of themselves and their abilities.*

*The conditions of empowerment were developed by Bonnie Benard, M.S.W., the founder of Resiliency Associates and the research editor of the journal *Resiliency in Action*.

Everyone—parents, teachers, community members—can support young people as they explore their inner and outer worlds.

Part of supporting our young people involves celebrating the transition from childhood to adulthood, the fact of becoming a woman or man. Our culture doesn't celebrate all that it means to be a woman—the substance of our minds, bodies, and spirits; the richness of our intellect, desires, and emotions. Women's bodies, with their curves of varying sizes, have great power: the power to attract and bear children, to dance and play sports. The female mind also possesses great power: the power to analyze and create, to lead and empathize. There is great power in us. Girls need help to find it in themselves.

### Advice to schools

Schools can help their students develop, not only in an intellectual sense but in a broader sense: they can help young people develop their concept of self, and their ability to think, feel, and act based on a grounded perception of the world around them. To achieve this goal, I recommend that schools do the following:

- Train teachers to use techniques designed to develop various aspects of students, not just the "masculine" part of their intellect. With techniques found in the educational processes of confluent education, holistic education, the Montessori method, the Waldorf method, and Native American education, teachers can help students develop their sense of awareness and responsibility as they move through their academic, social, and psychological worlds. Learning can be less didactic, more interactive and relational, more attuned to the innate intellectual curiosity of each student.

- Encourage teachers to create a learning atmosphere that is intellectually nurturing. That atmosphere would promote self-knowledge and an understanding of the ways we connect with one another in our world.
- Provide full-time school social workers to help young people develop their psychological as well as academic selves. Today's young people face so many issues that negatively influence their emotional and physical health: divorce, poverty, substance abuse, eating disorders, physical abuse, etc. Kids are less able to learn if their energies, minds, and feelings are focused on these troubling issues in their lives. Therefore the availability of a full-time school counselor would help kids not only emotionally but also academically.
- Train teachers to be aware of eating disorders and the steps they can take when they see a student with a problem. Schools tend to focus on kids who act out and cause problems in the school system, while students with eating disorders tend to succeed academically and cause problems for no one but themselves. Therefore teachers must be trained to notice the signs of eating disorders and act on those signs so students don't struggle in invisibility. With improved teacher awareness and the availability of on-site counselors, kids won't float through school without an anchor of support. They will be seen and heard and helped.
- Establish links with community resources so schools are part of a network for youth development.
- Work with educational researchers to take action based on scientifically sound research reports. By strengthening the link between the educational research community and schools, educational theory can be put into practice for the benefit of students. For example, an American Association of University Women report entitled *Shortchanging Girls,*

*Shortchanging America** shows that schools inadvertently discriminate against girls because teachers aren't trained to deal with the differing needs of males and females in the classroom. Based on this and other reports, schools can take specific steps to improve the learning environment for all students.

- In health or human development classes, discuss issues of sexuality; rather than promoting sex, such discussions can promote an understanding and acceptance of one's body and desires, an awareness of oneself, and a sense of responsibility for one's actions. In this environment, adolescents can discover that their sexuality is natural and beautiful, that sex and sexuality are different, and that an emerging sexuality doesn't indicate a readiness to have sex but instead might indicate a readiness to dance in front of a mirror, masturbate, write about desires, kiss.

- In health or human development classes, help students discover the importance of establishing emotional and psychological lives that are healthy for them.

- Establish after-school or in-school discussion groups for females and for males. Some of kids' needs are met through after-school programs like football, gymnastics, the student council, the school newspaper. But other basic adolescent needs often go unmet: the need to talk with one another in a safe space about the issues they are grappling with, and the need to process their feelings openly and nonjudgmentally. Some difficult and powerful issues faced by adolescents include sexuality, schoolwork, body image, drug use, violence, self-esteem, desire, fear, anger, and self-doubt. In safe spaces run by a counselor, young people of both genders

*The report can be obtained from the American Association of University Women in Washington, D.C. This report inspired Peggy Orenstein to write an engaging book entitled *Schoolgirls: Young Women, Self-esteem, and the Confidence Gap* (New York: Doubleday, 1994).

have the opportunity to find their voice and learn to listen. Occasionally the single-sex groups could come together to speak, listen, connect, and share.

### Advice to health care providers

If health care providers—doctors, nurses, dentists, gynecologists, pediatricians, etc.—are knowledgeable about eating disorders and are motivated to help girls and women, they can be an important resource for people with anorexia and bulimia. I recommend that concerned health care providers do the following:

- Educate yourselves about eating disorders: their causes, symptoms, and treatments.
- Be on the alert for patients who exhibit signs of eating disorders.
- Speak in a nonjudgmental, caring, and informational way with patients who exhibit signs of eating disorders. Help them understand that an eating disorder is a psychological problem that is manifested through physical behavior.
- Contact therapists who work with eating disorders patients, not only so you can refer patients in need of help, but so you can form working relationships with therapists on specific cases.
- Support psychotherapy, work with therapists on cases where psychological and physical problems interact, and accept the fact that psychological problems can't be fixed quickly, unlike some physical problems.
- In order to provide care for those in need, don't withhold health insurance from people with an eating disorder or some other preexisting condition. Although this recommendation has more to do with policymakers and health maintenance organization administrators, I address it to health care providers nonetheless.

*Advice to policymakers and others in government*

Policymakers and others in government—members of Congress, state legislators, governors, the President, the Health and Human Services Secretary, the Food and Drug Administration chair, the Surgeon General, the Education Secretary, and state cabinet officials in the health and education fields—can all have an impact on the prevention and treatment of eating disorders by creating needed change in the education and public health systems. I recommend the following:

- Provide adequate funding for schools so they have not only proper supplies, appropriate class sizes, and substantial teacher training/support, but also a full-time counselor on staff to deal with the myriad needs of America's young people.
- Fund research and teacher training in the areas of holistic education and educational processes that are not didactic and purely cognitive. With a holistic education, students can learn about math, science, history, literature, as well as their psychological and physical selves. This will help encourage students to become creative, capable, knowledgeable adults.
- Regarding sex education in schools, prioritize public health, not politics.
- Regulate the diet industry with the same intensity applied to regulation of the cigarette industry.
- Reform the health care system so that care is available and affordable to all. Our current system is the best in the world for the very few, merely adequate for others, and nonexistent or available only on a crisis basis for too many. Only bold reform of the health care system can provide the kind of care our citizens deserve.

*Advice to the media*

Of those involved in the mainstream media—those who create

the images of ourselves that we as a culture see—I ask the following:

- Present a more open, interesting, and real view of beauty.
- Step back to read the magazines you publish, look at the pictures you print, absorb the images you broadcast, and ask
yourself whether you are conveying a healthy and/or thought-
ful message.

### Advice to all community members

We can all play a role in helping young people develop their
desires, appetites, curiosity, intellect, creativity. We can help
them deal with the struggles they face not by providing answers,
but by listening, supporting, and caring. We can help them find
the compassion and strength to explore themselves and their
world. Specifically, you can:

- Support the creation of girls' groups in your community.*
- Help girls establish healthy rituals to deal with life's transi-
tions so they can give up such rituals as dieting and the
behaviors associated with eating disorders.
- Seek out and support alternative media outlets that offer views
of our culture, our world, and ourselves that differ from those
presented by the mainstream media. These outlets, which can
be found on magazine racks, at independent bookstores, on
the Web, and on television, recognize that beauty means more
than two-dimensional cookie-cutter images of thin models in
skimpy clothes. They recognize that beauty is three-dimen-
sional, reflecting individual style, ideas, feelings, experiences,
creativity, self-knowledge, compassion, and substance.
- Value children, teachers, social workers, therapists, and parents.
- Support some of the changes suggested in this chapter.

*See the Appendix for organizations involved in establishing girls' groups.

# T E N

■

# Advice to Parents, Siblings, Partners, Friends, and Mentors

YOUR role in helping a person with an eating disorder will vary depending on whether you are her mother, her sixteen-year-old friend, her student council adviser, her husband, etc. But whatever your relationship to her and whatever her age, you can best help a person with an eating disorder if you observe the signs of distress; approach her calmly, empathetically, and informationally; and help her reach her own decision to deal with her eating disorder and its underlying causes.

If a person you care about is struggling with an eating disorder, the signs will be all around you: panic or anger accompanying a break in a diet/exercise routine, secretive throwing-away of food, extreme and/or unnecessary weight loss, large fluctuations in weight, secretive eating of food accompanied by emotions like anger or sadness, "all or none" comments about weight such as "I didn't exercise for two days and now all I can wear is sweatpants because I look fat," etc. The signs of an eating disorder can be spotted without spying—without violating the person's trust and pushing her further into the isolation of her coping mechanism. If you make an effort to listen and become attuned to your daughter/friend/sister/etc., you will be able to determine whether she needs help for an eating disorder.

If you see signs of an eating disorder, I am urging you to gather your own strength and talk with the girl/woman, no matter how hard that might be for you. The following bullet points will help you through that talk, although they are not concrete steps that will lead to a quick remedy for a person's eating disorder. I would be dishonest if I claimed to know a definite and concrete path to change. Instead I am being honest with myself and with you by giving you guidelines, and hoping that you will trust yourself to examine these guidelines and hold them in your mind and body before talking with the girl/woman. Although the idea of approaching the girl/woman might be frightening for you, you will be able to talk with her. Each of us has instincts of caring and human kindness; when you trust those instincts, you will say what needs to be said in the moment.

- Prepare for the talk by reading about eating disorders in books, on the Web, and in materials provided by eating disorders organizations.* Learn about their causes, emotional and behavioral complexities, treatments, etc.
- Approach the girl/woman calmly when you are in a private space that is comfortable for both of you.
- Expect and accept that the girl/woman will most likely push you away when you approach her. Although she is rejecting you on the surface, she is absorbing your words and concern. You will need to approach her again once she has had a

---

*The contact information for various national eating disorders organizations is in the Appendix.

chance to reflect on your first discussion. Helping a person with an eating disorder is not a one-shot deal.

- Let her know you are talking with her not because she has done something wrong, but because you are seriously concerned about the way she is hurting herself physically and emotionally.
- Ask her what's wrong and listen to the answer without dismissing her concerns or expressing shame about her eating disorder.
- Focus on what she is feeling. Don't get stuck on issues of weight, body image, and dieting because the eating disorder, at its essence, isn't about those issues.
- Acknowledge the self-destructive eating behavior, but emphasize that the real problem is the deeper emotional struggle going on inside her.
- Recognize the importance of her coping mechanism to her—recognize that she will need that coping mechanism until she has established new ways to deal with herself in her world.
- Do not try to cure the eating disorder.
- Do not offer or accept quick fixes: diets are harmful, trips to Europe are diversionary. The only thing that will help is ongoing therapy.
- Let her know that dealing with an eating disorder is a long and sometimes frightening process, but that she can ask for whatever help she needs whenever she needs it.
- Recognize that your goal is to help her come to her own conclusion that she has the ability and desire to get help in the form of therapy.
- Gather the names of potential therapists who have experience in treating eating disorders. You can obtain the names of good therapists by asking a school counselor, your doctor, a local women's health center, one of the national eating disorders organizations, and/or people you

admire, respect, and trust. By getting the names of more than one therapist, you are letting her know that she has control over the therapy process, because she can shop around until she finds the therapist with whom she feels most comfortable.

• Offer to take her to a therapy session when she is ready.

You can follow these guidelines, express your concern for the girl/woman, and repeatedly offer her help, but you cannot fix her eating disorder—that's not a responsibility any of us can take for another person. Ultimately, she must make the decision to seek help for her own emotional, physical, and spiritual health.

### Advice specific to parents

By following the guidelines above, you will have a chance to reach your daughter and help her through the process of releasing herself from an eating disorder. However, since you are in a unique role as her parent, you have some additional responsibilities, many of which are difficult.

• Listen to another person if she/he notices signs of an eating disorder in your daughter. It is easy to dismiss another person's concerns, especially if you haven't noticed the signs yourself or have been afraid to act on them. But for the benefit of your daughter, you can use someone else's observations as an impetus to look for the signs and take action.

• Examine whether you are transmitting your own eating and body issues to your child by dieting, commenting on your own weight, commenting on other people's weight, etc. Without blaming you for your child's eating disorder, I am asking you to become conscious of your own relationship to food and body.

• Ask other people—people whom your daughter admires and

trusts—to speak with her, following the guidelines listed above. Sometimes a girl's mentor or older relative can reach her in a way you cannot. Your relationship with your daughter may be charged with negative emotions right now, while her relationship with a mentor is, most likely, charged with positive emotions. As a parent, you can use that resource to help your child.

- See a family therapist with your daughter and other family members. A family therapist can provide a safe space for family members to discuss issues they may not be able to address without a professional serving as a mediator, facilitator, and guide.* I want to emphasize that family therapy is not about blaming parents, it's about establishing a healthier dynamic for the whole family.

  Some parents might find the suggestion of family therapy threatening because it implies a change in the family system. It's true that parents may need to change the way they deal with emotions, listen to their child, handle a divorce, confront their own body issues, etc. And it's true that this notion can be frightening. I want to recognize the potential anger and fear that this suggestion may raise in some readers. Nonetheless, for the sake of girls with eating disorders, I make this statement and hope that parents will listen: parents should attend family therapy with their daughter.

- Enter into your own therapy if that is advised by the family therapist.

- Release some of your own concern, anger, sadness, and other emotions regarding your daughter's behavior by joining a support group for parents of children with eating disorders. For the sake of your own health as well as that of your daughter, you need to start dealing with the emotions the eating disorder creates in you.

*For a brief discussion of guidelines concerning how to choose a therapist, see page 161.

- As your daughter starts seeing a therapist—and, if necessary, a doctor working with the therapist to ensure that she isn't in immediate physical danger—you need to give your daughter space. I can understand your desire to help her get over the eating disorder immediately. But she doesn't need that pressure. She needs support, space, time, and love so she can go through her own process of healing. That process is arduous, frustrating, and filled with sadness, but it is the only path to freedom.

### Advice specific to friends, mentors, and siblings of a girl with an eating disorder

As someone who cares about a girl who is struggling with an eating disorder, your goal is to help that girl start the process of dealing with her eating disorder, either by helping her find a therapist she trusts, or by helping her start a discussion with her parents that will lead to therapy.

- If the girl is receptive to the idea of seeing a counselor but not to the idea of talking with her parents, support her in her effort to find a therapist she trusts. When she finds such a therapist, your main job is done. She and the therapist can discuss ways of involving the parents.
- If the girl is receptive to the idea of talking with her parents, let her know that you will help her by approaching her parents first, accompanying her when she approaches her parents, or otherwise serving as a support. If her parents are receptive to the idea of helping their daughter deal with her eating disorder, your main job is done.
- If the girl doesn't respond to your concern and suggestions after a couple of talks, let her know that you are approaching her parents. Talking with parents is a difficult matter, given that some may be defensive about what they perceive as a

judgment on their parenting skills. Explain to the parents that you are acting out of concern, not out of judgment; provide the parents with empathy and space so they can hear your message. Come prepared with the names of a few family therapists with experience in treating eating disorders. If the parents are receptive, you have accomplished your goal.

- If the parents are unreceptive, talk with the girl again to help her accept the idea of seeing a therapist. You can offer to go to a therapy session with her or talk with the therapist in advance. Once she finds a professional she connects with, you have accomplished your main goal. Now you can listen and provide support as needed. But the therapist is the person best able to deal with the girl's eating disorder, her crises, and the family's lack of support for counseling.

If you are the girl's peer, you too can offer support, provide information, help her talk with her parents, and encourage her to see a therapist. If you feel she won't take your concerns seriously, you may want to ask for help from one of the girl's mentors or from your own parents. Together, you and that person can go through the process described above. At the same time, you can provide the kind of support and comfort that can only come from a friend.

### Advice specific to partners of a woman with an eating disorder

As the partner of a woman with an eating disorder, you have some additional responsibilities for helping her let go.

- Emphasize that you love your partner—all of her—including her inner and outer beauty.
- Do not question her in a judgmental way about the food she eats or does not eat.
- Realize that the therapy process may affect your sex life.

Advice to Parents, Siblings, Partners, Friends, and Mentors

- Seek couples therapy to work through the effects of the eating disorder on you and the relationship.* Couples therapy can give the two of you a safe space to discuss and process issues you couldn't bring up without a professional mediator and facilitator.
- Remember that working through an eating disorder is a long and difficult process. Your patience and love is a great support for your partner.

*For a brief discussion of guidelines concerning how to choose a therapist, see page 161.

# E L E V E N

·

# Advice to Girls and Women Experiencing an Eating Disorder

THROUGH this book, I have shared part of my journey with you. Through this last chapter, I hope to help you on your own journey toward feeling and experiencing the whole of yourself.

The process of change starts with the desire for change—the desire to experience more than the eating disorder will allow. If you are not sure that you feel the desire to change yet—if you feel uncertain or threatened by the thought of living without your eating disorder—I want you to know that I respect your position, because I have been there, too. I have heard my body scream, "STOP! NO! I'm not giving up my eating disorder! I'm not listening to talk about treatment!" I have no intention of *making* you listen to talk about treatment, but I hope to make it *easier* for you to listen. Getting help doesn't mean that someone is criticizing you, taking control away from you, telling you to give up your coping mechanism before you are ready. Getting help means that you are making the choice to grow for your own health and freedom and life.

Before describing specific therapies for the treatment of eating disorders, I want to acknowledge some common obstacles to seeking help and introduce some basic ideas about therapy.

Each of the following obstacles is valid and large and looming. And each can be dealt with, given time and care. Shame is a natural obstacle to treatment, given that we hide our behavior and are fearful of the judgments of others. But facing that shame is an important part of the process of letting go. After ten years of struggling with an eating disorder, I realized that people with anorexia and bulimia have nothing to be ashamed of: we are strong to have found a way to survive when we weren't offered the support we needed. At some point, you will probably come to a similar realization, and will begin to focus your energy on changing rather than hiding.

Along with shame, fear prevents many of us from seeking treatment: fear of losing our identity and fear of existing without our coping mechanism. Once you have relied on an eating disorder, you can lose the sense of who you are without it—without that part of you that has defined so much of your thinking and being: Will I lose my intensity, my deep emotions? Will I lose the ability to be thin—the only thing that makes me stand apart? Will I lose my pathology, my label of someone with a problem? Who am I then? This fear of losing one's identity is palpable and real. When you start therapy, you and your therapist can discuss ways of helping you overcome it. Your therapist can also help as you deal with the fear of living without your eating disorder. That fear will start to dissolve as you discover new ways to handle the powerful emotions and experiences that led you to develop an eating disorder in the first place.

Fear can be exacerbated by another common obstacle to getting help: a lack of family support. Ideally, when you seek treatment for an eating disorder, you will not be doing so alone.

Ideally, your parents will also seek treatment in an effort to understand their role in the development of the eating disorder and to change unhealthy family dynamics. But such ideal circumstances aren't real for too many of us. If your family is actively against therapy for you, you'll need the support of a friend, mentor, advocate, school counselor, caring adult, etc., who can help you get treatment. If you start getting treatment, you are not betraying your family, you are taking care of yourself. A good therapist will work with you to help you deal with the resistance of your parents.

Finally, it's easy to avoid therapy when you don't know what to expect, where to look, whom to talk to, what to ask. The remainder of this chapter is intended to help you gain that knowledge in a comprehensive way.

The following are some basic ideas concerning the treatment process. Treatment will be easier if you keep these ideas in mind as you move along in the process of letting go.

- Therapy isn't about being weak or crazy or unsuccessful. It is about being strong enough to realize that you need help in finding ways to experience all of yourself.
- Treatment is work. I don't want to underplay the slow, difficult, and frustrating nature of treatment, because I don't want you to quit before you have gotten what you need. So I am urging you to hold on to the knowledge that although treatment is arduous, it is your one path to freedom.
- Part of the frustration of treatment is the inevitable "slipping back" into old behaviors. I want you to understand that both progress and "relapse" are part of letting go. And I hope you can forgive yourself when you experience a relapse.
- There is no "right" therapy combination. You must choose among the therapies and decide which ones will best help *you* heal. Your choice is never irreversible: you can always add some therapies and drop others to find what works for

you. As you read the next pages, you might try to notice which therapies cause a positive reaction in you—which engage your curiosity, ease your anxiety, stimulate your imagination. Then you will have a starting point for therapy.

- Individual psychotherapy is the only type of therapy that *all* people with an eating disorder should have as part of their treatment. It is the most effective means of long-term change.
- While everyone with an eating disorder should have the help of an individual psychotherapist, not every psychotherapist should help someone with an eating disorder. Part of me is wary of sending all readers off to therapy, because I know that there are many therapists who are not trained to deal with the emotional and physical issues surrounding an eating disorder. But another part of me knows that you can only get better by finding good professional help. That's why it is vital for you to choose a therapist with whom you are comfortable, and to shop around until you find that therapist.
- Therapy takes time and money, but you are worth the sacrifice. This is the most important investment you can make.
- Treatment means growth, and growth means change. Therefore, letting go of an eating disorder will entail major changes in the way you relate to yourself, to your body, to other people, and to the world around you.
- In order to be effective, treatment must be holistic, meaning that it must address all aspects of your being—your mind, body, and spirit, as well as the flow among the three.
- The best way to approach the treatment of your eating disorder is on three levels: medically, psychologically, and spiritually.

### *The beginning step in eating disorders treatment: The medical level*

The first step in seeking help is to get a good medical exam from a doctor who has had experience working with eating dis-

orders patients. Eating disorders can have serious medical com-
plications that a doctor can diagnose and treat. When you see
the doctor, let her/him know about your history with anorexia
and/or bulimia. Ask that person if she/he has had experience
treating eating disorders or can refer you to a doctor who does.
You might want to ask a family member, friend, counselor,
mentor, etc., to lend support and comfort by accompanying
you to the doctor's office.

While most people with eating disorders do not have urgent
medical conditions, some of us are medically compromised and
need to be stabilized. This is most common among people who
are severely anorexic. If you are in that situation, I recommend
that you enter the medical unit of a hospital with the sole purpose of getting to the point of medical safety, not with the purpose of ending your eating disorder. If you enter a hospital, you
should ask to see a therapist who can be your advocate, help
you through the frightening hospitalization, and work with the
medical doctor.

If you feel a short hospitalization is insufficient for helping you to become medically stabilized, I recommend that
you enter a twenty-eight-day residential program designed
for people with eating disorders. These programs can provide a time-out from your behavior, help establish medical
stabilization, and prepare you physically and emotionally for
the hard work involved in long-term therapy. But these programs cannot cure your eating disorder. You should not
enter them for any reason other than the opportunity for a
time-out and for help in getting medically stabilized.
Despite the comfort and support they provide, these programs are disappointing and ineffective in terms of creating
deep change.

If your medical condition is not urgent or has been stabilized, you can begin working regularly with a therapist to deal
with the psychological and spiritual issues surrounding the eat-

ing disorder. That therapist should keep in contact with your doctor in order to monitor your medical condition.

### The longest step in eating disorders treatment: The psychological level

Once you have consulted a doctor and explored the medical side of treatment, you can begin to contact therapists that specialize in eating disorders. You can locate different therapists by asking people you trust, your school mental-health counselor, the local women's health center, your doctor, or one of the national eating disorders organizations.* I recommend that you get the names of several therapists so you have control over determining the person you will be working with, and can shop around until you find a therapist who fits your needs.

You will know which therapist fits your needs by acting on instinct—on what feels right. You may want to ask yourself certain questions: Do I feel I am being judged by the therapist? Does she/he understand the behaviors and emotional issues I am grappling with? Do I feel comfortable talking with her/him? If you find a therapist you immediately connect with, your decision is easy. But if you are uncertain after the initial meeting, I suggest seeing that therapist at least one more time, as well as seeing another therapist to get a feel for someone else's style. Eventually, you will find the person who is right for you.

A long-term **individual psychotherapy** relationship with a therapist experienced in the treatment of eating disorders is the one effective, long-lasting form of eating disorders therapy. This trusting and compassionate environment can become your "therapeutic container." By allowing your therapist to contain the burden of your emotions, you can follow her/his guidance

*The contact information for various national eating disorders organizations is in the Appendix.

and begin reexamining your assumptions, patterns, and perceptions. The therapeutic container can give you some emotional breathing room—some space and time and relief—so you can work on making changes and developing a new relationship to yourself (including the parts of you that have been hurt or undeveloped), other people, and the world around you.

I strongly recommend **family therapy** if you are living at home. Since you would not have developed an eating disorder if your family atmosphere were completely healthy, you and your parents should attend therapy together. Some parents think only their daughter needs help, and will refuse to enter family therapy. That refusal often arises because they cannot handle the idea of embarking on their own psychological work and making deep changes within themselves. If you are in that situation, you can work with your therapist to establish a relationship with your parents that gives you the distance you need to be able to grow. It will be difficult, but it is worth it—you are worth it.

If you are in a stable and serious relationship, I recommend **couples therapy**. In couples therapy, both partners can establish new ways of relating to each other and to their world, and can process the emotions surrounding the eating disorder and its underlying causes.

Some of you will benefit from **group therapy**, in which approximately five to fifteen people get together with a therapist to share their problems, concerns, feelings, and solutions. In group therapy, participants can experience a feeling of community and empathy, develop skills in relating to other people, and explore how to deal with a culture that negatively influences women's views of their bodies and themselves.

In some cases, the most effective treatment is the use of **antidepressants** in conjunction with individual psychotherapy. Not everyone with an eating disorder needs to be on an antidepressant; I suggest that you first try individual psychotherapy alone.

But some of us have a fundamental biochemical imbalance that is linked to the depression or anxiety underlying the eating disorder. If you feel suicidal or unable to function, do not hesitate to talk with your therapist about antidepressants.

As previously discussed, antidepressants help regulate mood by regulating neurotransmitter levels. By easing anxiety and reducing urgency, antidepressants can give people the psychological space needed to be able to experience and deal with their problems. But the medication alone is not enough: an antidepressant is simply a tool that allows the hard work of therapy to progress without being crushed at each step by depression, obsessiveness, anxiety, etc.

If you take an antidepressant, you are not forever dependent on it. Once you have established new patterns while on the antidepressant—often after a year or two—you can start to implement those new patterns without the medication. In addition, you can always get off the medication if it makes you uncomfortable. The newest class of antidepressants—selective serotonin reuptake inhibitors (SSRIs)—have fewer side effects than previous antidepressants, and are therefore more useful in helping people with clinical diagnoses like depression, anorexia, or bulimia. However, SSRIs, like all medications, can have side effects, depending on the individual and the brand of the antidepressant. These side effects can often be alleviated or eliminated by working with a psychiatrist or doctor to change the brand or type of antidepressant or to adjust the dosage.

When you are deciding whether to take the medication, talk with your therapist about any concerns you have. You should not be forced to take an antidepressant. It is your choice.

**Expressive therapies**, such as art and drama therapy, allow us to communicate in nonverbal ways and articulate emotions that we don't yet have words for. If you were in art therapy, you would be asked to draw a feeling or situation. The pictures drawn—for example, a tiny person in the corner of the page with a man looming large above her — can reveal emotions that couldn't yet be expressed through words. If you were in drama therapy, you would be asked to act out an emotion or scenario. By "acting," you may be able to get outside yourself and express feelings you might otherwise keep bottled up inside you. Once the emotions or situations come to the surface through expressive therapies, you and the therapist can examine and deal with them. Although expressive therapies use drawing and acting as therapeutic tools, clients do not need artistic skill to participate in them.

Expressive therapies are sometimes conducted by individual psychotherapists, and sometimes conducted by therapists who run groups specifically focused on expressive therapies. If you think expressive therapies might be helpful for you, talk with your primary therapist about whether she/he is experienced in those techniques. If not, ask her/him if she/he knows a therapist who runs an expressive therapy group and would be willing to collaborate with you and your primary therapist.

**Active imagination, guided imagery, and other forms of hypnotherapy** can also allow you to examine your emotions without the interference of your mind. Through these techniques, you can be led into a highly relaxed state in which you can experience yourself moving through various situations and their accompanying feelings. You and your therapist can later talk about the images that emerge, and the intensity and realness of the feelings that arise. These techniques, combined with therapist-client discussion, can help create a sense of empathy, connection, resolution, and clarity regarding ways you can deal with uncomfortable situations. Despite the somewhat shady reputation of hypnotherapy, control of the situation will never be taken from you if you are working with an experienced and moral therapist.

However, these techniques must be applied within the context of an established therapy relationship. They are dangerous if applied by someone who has not worked with you before, and who does not have a long-term therapist-client relationship with you. I strongly recommend that you only undergo these techniques if your primary therapist is trained as a hypnotherapist, and if you are working regularly with her/him.

While you deal with the deeper issues underlying the eating disorder, you will also need specific tools to help you deal with the actual eating behavior and the daily issues you face as a person with anorexia or bulimia. The technique of **cognitive behavioral therapy** (CBT) involves using your cognition/mind to notice the thoughts and actions that trigger and surround both your eating behavior and your negative feelings toward yourself. When you have started noticing your patterns, you and your therapist can work toward developing alternative ways to deal with your cravings and your judgments about your worth as a person.

In order to complete the process of healing, you must work specifically on reconnecting with your body through **body work** like yoga, tai chi, shiatsu, massage therapy, exercise, etc. Eastern-based body work like yoga, tai chi, and shiatsu seeks to restore the natural flow of the body and to connect people with their body's healing energy. These principles also form the basis of massage therapy, in which a trained therapist manipulates your muscle tissues in order to induce relaxation and increase the removal of toxins from your body. Through various forms of exercise like dance, walking, biking, swimming, etc., you may start to feel your body working in a positive way, generating energy, using its power as it was meant to. Some people may enjoy aerobics classes, weight training, or jogging. But I would caution against exercise that feeds into an eating disorder and the use of body manipulation for purposes of psychological relief. Therefore some of you may want to temporarily avoid "hard-core" exercise and those forms of exercise that you have used as part of your eating disorder. Instead you might benefit from other types of exercise until you feel you are no longer obsessive in this realm.

At a certain stage of your treatment, you need to **become attuned to your body's nutritional needs**. When your nutritional intake is balanced, your body can more easily avoid the impulses that sustain an eating disorder. To help you restore nutritional balance, you can work with your therapist in keeping a food journal where you will record what you eat and when, as well as what you feel before, during, and after you eat. In doing so, you will notice patterns relating to your eating behavior. By examining those patterns with a therapist, you can begin to develop techniques to help change that behavior.

The one sure way *not* to connect with your body in a healthy way is through dieting. Diets might help you lose some weight, and maybe you will even keep it off. For a few days. Maybe even for a few weeks. But if you follow one of the popular regimented diets, you are not going to establish a positive relationship with yourself and your body, and you are going to undermine the healthy, beautiful body that you are meant to have by nature.

### The ultimate and most long-lasting step in eating disorders treatment: The spiritual level

The ultimate goal of eating disorders treatment is to develop yourself spiritually. When I say this, I do not mean that the goal is to develop connections to a religion or "God." Rather, the goal is to develop meaningful connections with yourself, with others, and with the world around you, as well as an understanding of the interconnectedness among the three.

It is difficult to grow spiritually when you have an eating disorder—when you are creating a wall between yourself and your emotions, and between yourself and other people. As therapy helps you dissolve these walls, you will begin to experience the full range of your feelings and your self. You can taste more of life by exploring different emotions, experiences, people, and situations. Writing in a journal, creating music, painting, volunteering, being in nature, opening yourself to another person . . . I can't name all the ways toward spiritual development, because there is no end to them. Your ways are to be discovered and rediscovered always.

RELEASING YOURSELF FROM an eating disorder is not a linear process. There aren't twelve steps you must walk to get to the finish line. Instead there is your own path with dead ends and steep climbs, nurturing air and luscious fruits. Everything you do in life is part of the path that you create for yourself, and everything you do will enrich your experience. No matter how much it seems like there's only one way, there are more; no matter how monolithic your community seems, there are people with values, desires, and perceptions similar to yours, and you can find them.

Everyone's path is different. The path I've made has led me here. I have more territory to cover — both in my internal and external world — and I will explore my growing path. You will explore yours, too. At some point you will look back and see part of that path — the swamp you climbed from, the lake you floated over, the trees you leaned on, the people who gave you strength.

As I write these last lines, I feel like our paths have crossed. Even though we haven't met and we haven't talked face-to-face, our paths have crossed. And before we leave each other, I want you to know that throughout me — throughout my mind and body and spirit — I hope you find more forgiving and supportive terrain. Feel yourself. See yourself. Know your power. Good luck on your journey.

# A P P E N D I X

∎

# Where to Find What
# You Need

## Eating Disorders: National Organizations

American Anorexia/Bulimia Association (AABA)
165 West 46th Street, Suite 1108
New York, NY 10036
(212) 575-6200
Web site: http://members.aol.com/AMANBU
• Provides referrals, nationwide
• Runs support groups
• Maintains a speakers' bureau, nationwide
• Conducts educational outreach

Center for the Study of Anorexia and Bulimia (CSAB)
1841 Broadway
New York, NY 10023
(212) 595-3449; fax: (212) 333-5444
• Provides referrals, nationwide
• Conducts educational outreach: speaking engagements, workshops, reading lists, lecture series
• Runs a training program for professionals who want specialization
in treating eating disorders

Eating Disorders Awareness & Prevention (EDAP)
603 Stewart Street, Suite 803
Seattle, WA 98101
(206) 382-3587; fax: (206) 292-9890
Web site: http://members.aol.com/edapinc
• Provides educational materials: curricula, educational programs, videos, newsletter, conferences, workshops
• Sponsors the National Eating Disorders Awareness Week each February
• Maintains a speakers' bureau, nationwide

International Association of Eating Disorders Professionals
123 NW 13th Street, #206
Boca Raton, FL 33432
(561) 338-6494; fax: (561) 338-9913
Web site: http://www.iaedp.com
• Provides certification and training for eating disorders professionals
• Provides referrals, nationwide
• Maintains a speakers' bureau, nationwide

Massachusetts Eating Disorders Association (MEDA)
92 Pearl Street
Newton, MA 02158
(617) 558-1818; fax: (617) 558-1771
Web site: http://www.medainc.org
• Runs support groups for people with eating disorders, parents, and friends and family
• Provides referrals, mainly in Massachusetts
• Conducts educational outreach: curriculum development, seminars for schools from preschool to college

National Association of Anorexia Nervosa and Associated Disorders (ANAD)
Box 7
Highland Park, IL 60035
(847) 831-3438; fax: (847) 433-4632; e-mail: anad20@aol.com
Web site: http://www.healthtouch.com
• Provides referrals, nationwide and internationally
• Provides referrals for support groups, nationwide
• Maintains a hot line staffed by counselors
• Provides educational materials: information packets, Web site

National Eating Disorder Information Centre (NEDIC)
College Wing 1-211
200 Elizabeth Street
Toronto, ON M5G 2C4
Canada
(416) 340-4156
- Provides referrals, nationwide
- Provides referrals for support groups, nationwide
- Conducts educational outreach: information packets, prevention and treatment campaigns, lectures and workshops for schools, community groups, and professionals

International Eating Disorders Organization (NEDO)
6655 South Yale Avenue
Tulsa, OK 74136
(918) 481-4044; fax: (918) 481-4076
Web site: http://www.laureate.com
- Provides referrals, nationwide and internationally
- Provides referrals for support groups, nationwide
- Provides educational materials: information packets, information phone line, curricula

When you explore the Web sites listed above, you will find links to various other eating disorder Web sites; many of them are well worth looking through. You can also check out various news groups on eating disorders. Unlike Web sites, news groups allow participants to read and share messages with other news-group participants. Of all the eating disorder news groups, alt.support.eating-disord.com seems to be the most active and informative.

## OTHER HELPFUL ORGANIZATIONS

Girls' Circle
6 Knoll Lane, Suite F
Mill Vally, CA 94941
(415) 388-0644
- Runs workshops to train adults how to run girls' support groups
- Provides educational materials: training manual, facilitator's guide to running girls' groups

Appendix

Girls Speak Out
P.O. Box 1799
Guerneville, CA 95446
(707) 869-0829
• Runs consciousness-raising programs for girls ages 9 to 16
• Runs a global girls' political action network

Girls Incorporated
30 East 33rd Street
New York, NY 10016-5394
(212) 689-3700; fax: (212) 683-1253
Web site: http://www.girlsinc.org
• Sponsors research-based educational programs for girls
• Serves 350,000 young people, ages 6 to 18, at over 1,000 sites nationwide

The Ophelia Project
2729 Exposition Boulevard, Box 192
Austin, TX 78703
(512) 476-3988; fax: (512) 476-3911
• Provides up-to-date information about girls' self-esteem needs; speakers' series in schools, workshops, and conferences
• Advocates for girls' needs in schools, communities, and the media

Resiliency in Action
P.O. Box 684
Gorham, ME 04038
(505) 323-1031; fax: (505) 323-1582
Web site: http://www.resiliency.com
• Publishes the journal *Resiliency in Action: A National Journal of Resiliency Application and Practical Research*
• Runs trainings, seminars, and conferences